Managing Obesity and Eating Disorders

First Edition

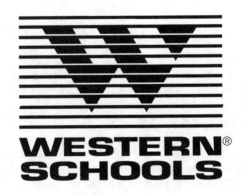

WESTERN® SCHOOLS

By
Nancy J. Gustafson, MS, RD, FADA

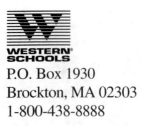

P.O. Box 1930
Brockton, MA 02303
1-800-438-8888

ABOUT THE AUTHOR

Nancy J. Gustafson, MS, RD, FADA is a registered dietitian, charter fellow of the American Dietetic Association, and freelance medical writer. She has authored or co-authored four books and numerous professional articles on nutrition and health. As clinical dietitian at Carle Clinic in Urbana, Illinois, she specialized in management of obesity and eating disorders.

Copy Editor: Becky Colgan

Indexer: Sylvia Coates

Typesetter: Kathy Johnson

ISBN: 1-57801-007-1

IMPORTANT: Read these instructions *BEFORE* proceeding!

Enclosed with your course book you will find the FasTrax answer sheet. Use this form to answer all the final exam questions that appear in this course book. If you are completing more than one course, be sure to write your answers on the appropriate answer sheet. You have the option of faxing the FasTrax answer sheet to 508-230-2679 and within 48 hours get your course results automatically faxed back to you or you may elect to mail the FasTrax answer sheet to Western Schools and get your course results within 7–12 business days. Full instructions and complete grading details are also printed on the FasTrax instruction sheet, please review them before starting. *If you are mailing your answer sheets to Western Schools, we recommend you make a xerox copy as a backup.*

ABOUT THIS COURSE

A "Pretest" is provided with each course to test your current knowledge base regarding the subject matter contained within this course. Your "Final Exam" is a multiple choice examination. **You will find the exam questions at the end of each chapter.**

In the event the course has less than 100 questions, leave the remaining answer boxes on the FasTrax answer sheet blank.

A PASSING SCORE

You must score 70% or better in order to pass this course and receive your Certificate of Completion. Should you fail to achieve the required score, we will send you an additional FasTrax answer sheet so that you may make a second attempt to pass the course. Western Schools will allow you three chances to pass the same course…*at no extra charge!* After three failed attempts to pass the same course, your file will be closed.

RECORDING YOUR HOURS

Please monitor the time it takes to complete this course using the handy log sheet on the other side of this page. See below for transferring study hours to the course evaluation.

On the back of the FasTrax instruction sheet there is additional space to make any comments about the course, the school, and suggested new curriculum. Please mail the FasTrax instruction sheet back to Western Schools in the envelope provided with your course order.

COURSE EVALUATIONS

In this course book you will find a short evaluation about the course you are soon to complete. This information is vital to providing the school with feedback on this course. The course evaluation answer section is in the lower right hand corner of the FasTrax answer sheet marked "Evaluation" with answers marked 1–25. Your answers are important to us, please take five minutes to complete the evaluation. Thank you.

TRANSFERRING STUDY TIME

Upon completion of the course, transfer the total study time from your log sheet to question #25 in the Course Evaluation. The answers will be in ranges, please choose the proper hour range that best represents your study time. You MUST log your study time under question #25 on the course evaluation.

EXTENSIONS

You have 2 years from the date of enrollment to complete this course. A six (6) month extension may be purchased for $25. If after 30 months from the original enrollment date you do not complete the course, *your file will be closed and no certificate can be issued.*

CHANGE OF ADDRESS?

In the event you have moved during the completion of this course please call our student services department at 1-800-618-1670 and we will update your file.

NO RISK GUARANTEE

All Western Schools courses are backed by a No Risk Money Back Guarantee. If you're not satisfied with the quality of the course materials, you can return them unmarked within 30 days for a full refund (less shipping and handling). This does not apply to software courses.

Western Schools guarantees you will receive credit for this course from your state board or regulatory agency, or we will give you a full refund.

Thank you for enrolling at Western Schools!

WESTERN SCHOOLS
21 Bristol Drive, South Easton, MA 02375
(800) 438-8888
www.westernschools.com

Managing Obesity
and Eating Disorders

WESTERN® SCHOOLS
P.O. Box 1930
Brockton, MA 02303

Please use this log to total the number of hours you spend reading the text and taking the final examination (use 50-min hours).

Date	Hours Spent
————	————
————	————
————	————
————	————
————	————
————	————
————	————
————	————
————	————
————	————
————	————
————	————
————	————

TOTAL ☐

Please log your study hours with submission of your final exam. To log your study time, fill in the appropriate circle under question 25 of the FasTrax® answer sheet under the "Evaluation" section.

Please choose the answer that represents the total study hours it took you to complete this 30 hour course.

A. less than 25 hours   C. 29–32 hours

B. 25–28 hours   D. greater than 32 hours

Managing Obesity
and Eating Disorders

WESTERN SCHOOLS
CONTINUING EDUCATION EVALUATION

Instructions: Mark your answers to the following questions with a black pen on the "Evaluation" section of your FasTrax® answer sheet provided with this course. You should not return this sheet. Please use the scale below to rate the following statements:

A   Agree Strongly   **C   Disagree Somewhat**
B   Agree Somewhat   **D   Disagree Strongly**

The course content met the following education objectives

1. Identified new trends and issues in both ends of the weight management spectrum.

2. Recognized factors that influence body weight regulation and the development of obesity and eating disorders.

3. Identified health implications of obesity, weight loss, weight regain, and eating disorders.

4. Differentiated between normal weight, overweight, obesity, and eating disorders.

5. Described the key elements of a comprehensive assessment of patients with obesity or eating disorders.

6. Indicated appropriate therapy options for patients with varying degrees of obesity, eating disorders, and medical risk.

7. Recognized the components of a healthy and nutritionally adequate eating plan.

8. Identified the types and characteristics of conservative management approaches for obesity.

9. Described the types of aggressive interventions used for management of obesity.

10. Recognized the key components of nutritional management of patients with anorexia nervosa or bulimia nervosa.

11. Recognized the unique dietary management considerations for special groups of patients with obesity or eating disorders.

12. Identified the benefits of regular physical activity and specified reasonable guidelines for exercising safely for individuals with obesity or eating disorders.

13. Identified the factors that help patients achieve life-long changes for weight maintenance.

14. This offering met my professional education needs.

15. The information in this offering is relevant to my professional work setting.

16. The course was generally well written and the subject matter explained thoroughly? (If no please explain on the back of the FasTrax instruction sheet.)

17. The content of this course was appropriate for home study.

18. The final examination was well written and at an appropriate level for the content of the course.

Please complete the following research questions in order to help us better meet your educational needs. Pick the ONE answer which is most appropriate.

19. Do you usually exceed the contact hours required for your state license renewal, if so, why?

    A. Yes, I have more than one state license

    B. Yes, to meet additional special association Continuing Education requirements

    C. Yes, for professional self-interest/cross-training

    D. No, I only take the state required minimum

20. What nursing shift do you most commonly work?

    A. Morning Shift (Any shift starting after 3:00am or before 11:00am)

    B. Day/Afternoon Shift (Any shift starting after 11:00am or before 7:00pm)

    C. Night Shift (Any shift starting after 7:00pm or before 3:00am)

    D. I work rotating shifts

21. What was the SINGLE most important reason you chose this course?

    A. Low Price

    B. New or Newly revised course

    C. High interest/Required course topic

    D. Number of Contact Hours Needed

22. Where do you work? (If your place of employment is not listed below, please leave this question blank.)

    A. Hospital

    B. Medical Clinic/Group Practice/ HMO/Office setting

    C. Long Term Care/Rehabilitation Facility/Nursing Home

    D. Home Health Care Agency

23. Which field do you specialize in?

    A. Medical/Surgical

    B. Geriatrics

    C. Pediatrics/Neonatal

    D. Other

24. For your last renewal, how many months BEFORE your license expiration date did you order your course materials?

    A. 1–3 months

    B. 4–6 months

    C. 7–12 months

    D. Greater than 12 months

25. **PLEASE LOG YOUR STUDY HOURS WITH SUBMISSION OF YOUR FINAL EXAM.** Please choose which best represents the total study hours it took to complete this 30 hour course.

    A. less than 25 hours

    B. 25–28 hours

    C. 29–32 hours

    D. greater than 32 hours

CONTENTS

PRETEST

Begin by taking the pretest. Compare your answers on the pretest to the answer key (located in the back of the book). Circle those test items that you missed. The pretest answer key indicates the course chapters where the content of that question is discussed.

Next, read each chapter. Focus special attention on the chapters where you made incorrect answer choices. Exam questions are provided at the end of each chapter so that you can assess your progress and understanding of the material.

1. Obesity is considered a chronic disease because

   a. being obese permanently alters health status, regardless of whether or not the individual eventually loses weight.

   b. the incidence of obesity across all populations is rapidly rising.

   c. control of complex biological and environmental forces regulating body weight requires life-long vigilance.

   d. many of the health problems associated with obesity are chronic conditions.

2. Which of the following is similar in both obese patients and in patients with an eating disorder?

   a. physiological mechanisms regulating hunger, satiety, and body weight

   b. physiological regulation of thermogenesis

   c. psychological response to restrictive dieting, hunger, or starvation

   d. environmental stimulus control

3. Patients will gain weight if

   a. energy intake increases by 10 percent

   b. physical activity decreases by 10 percent

   c. energy intake chronically exceeds energy expenditure

   d. energy expenditure chronically exceeds energy intake

4. Men burn calories more quickly than women because

   a. they exercise more.

   b. they have more muscle tissue than women.

   c. they have more self-control than women.

   d. they have more fat tissue than women.

5. Obesity is a major risk factor in which leading cause of death in Americans?

   a. non-insulin-dependent diabetes

   b. suicide

   c. pneumonia and influenza

   d. chronic liver disease

6. Which of the following is an obesity-related risk factor for cardiovascular disease?

   a. type A personality

   b. high HDL cholesterol levels

   c. insulin-dependent diabetes mellitus

   d. high blood pressure

7. Body fat can be indirectly measured using which of the following

   a. underwater weighing

   b. bioelectrical impedance

   c. weight-for-height tables

   d. total body electrical conductivity

8. Excess fat deposits located in which area of the body are most associated with increased health risks?

    a. upper-chest area

    b. abdominal area ✓

    c. buttocks

    d. thighs

9. Which of the following are factors that would preclude initiating a weight control program?

    a. Patient just finished breast-feeding a child.

    b. Patient is a child.

    c. Patient is an older adult.

    d. Patient has a history of anorexia nervosa.

10. Which of the following is a physical sign of good nutrition?

    a. rapid heart rate

    b. brittle hair

    c. pale conjunctivas in eyes

    d. reddish-pink mucous membranes in oral cavity

11. One element of a successful weight management program is

    a. individualization ✓

    b. rapid weight loss

    c. strict control

    d. standardized meal plans

12. The ultimate goal of obesity management programs is

    a. slow but steady weight loss

    b. permanent weight maintenance

    c. a long-term energy deficit

    d. achieving desirable body weight

13. How many calories does one gram of fat contain?

    a. 3

    b. 4

    c. 7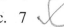

    d. 9 ✓

14. Which of the following should be consumed in greatest quantities and provide the foundation of a healthy diet in the Food Guide Pyramid?

    a. meat, poultry, fish, dry beans, eggs, and nuts

    b. vegetables

    c. breads, cereals, rice, and pasta ✓

    d. fruits

15. A calorie deficit of how many calories will lead to a weight loss of one pound?

    a. 2,000

    b. 3,500

    c. 5,000

    d. 7,500

16. Most inactive women maintain weight on about how many calories daily?

    a. 1,200 to 1,400

    b. 1,500 to 1,600

    c. 1,800 to 2,000 ✓

    d. 2,200 to 2,400

17. Aggressive management approaches may be appropriate for which group of patients?

    a. Patients 10 percent or more over ideal body weight who have obesity-related health problems.

    b. Patients 20 percent or more over ideal body weight who have obesity-related health problems.

    c. Patients 40 or more percent over ideal body weight who have obesity-related health problems.

    d. Patients who tried and failed to achieve significant weight loss using very low-calorie diets.

18. Low-calorie diets usually provide what number of calories daily?

    a. less than 500

    b. 500 to 800

    c. 800 to 1,200

    d. 1,200 or more

19. The lower the calorie content of the diet, the

    a. lower the carbohydrate content should be

    b. lower the protein content should be

    c. lower the fat content should be

    d. higher the fat content should be

20. Which of the following health professionals might be involved in carrying out a nutritional care plan?

    a. dietitians

    b. physicians

    c. nurses

    d. all of the above

21. One trend in management of patients with eating disorders is to provide more treatment

    a. on an outpatient basis

    b. on an inpatient basis

    c. in the patient's own home

    d. via the Internet

22. About what percent of sodium in the diet of Americans occurs naturally in foods?

    a. one-tenth

    b. one-quarter

    c. one-third

    d. one-half

23. Obesity appears to increase the risk of developing which types of cancer?

    a. lung

    b. breast

    c. bone

    d. skin

24. Physical activity has been shown to help prevent or treat which of the following chronic diseases?

    a. high blood pressure

    b. osteoporosis

    c. heart disease

    d. all of the above

25. Which takes longer to change in the patient with an eating disorder?

    a. nutritional status

    b. weight deficit

    c. food-related behavior

    d. thoughts and feelings about body image and food

CHAPTER 1

WEIGHT MANAGEMENT: A NEW AND INTEGRATED APPROACH

CHAPTER OBJECTIVE

After reading this chapter, you will be able to identify new trends and issues in both ends of the weight management spectrum.

LEARNING OBJECTIVES

After studying this chapter, you will be able to

1. Recognize why obesity must be viewed as a chronic disease.

2. Identify common issues in the management of obesity and eating disorders.

3. Specify trends in the prevalence of obesity and eating disorders.

4. Indicate new areas of focus for weight management approaches.

INTRODUCTION

At any one time, tens of millions of people in the United States are dieting. In fact, almost one-half of Americans consider themselves overweight. Americans spend over $33 million yearly in pursuit of thinness, and the health care industry spends another $70 billion treating obesity-related health problems of Americans. Diet programs and products continue to proliferate at a rapid rate.

Yet with all the effort directed toward attaining thinness, Americans on average are gaining, not losing, weight. The incidence of obesity is reaching epidemic proportions in the United States. In the early 1960s, 24 percent of Americans were considered overweight. Today about 35 percent of adult women in the United States and 31 percent of adult men are overweight. Even more alarming, almost 25 percent of children and teenagers in the United States are overweight.

For those individuals who do manage to lose weight, long-term statistics are bleak. Most individuals regain two-thirds of the weight loss within the first year after dieting and all or more of the weight loss within five years of dieting.

Amid America's weight obsession and the tremendous cultural pressures to be thin, eating disorders are also on the rise. Many individuals set themselves up for failure by striving to attain unrealistic weight goals. About 2 percent of females in the United States have serious forms of eating disorders such as anorexia nervosa and bulimia nervosa. About 10 percent of females have milder or variant versions of these eating disorders. Although much less common, the incidence of eating disorders among males is also increasing. Among individuals seeking to lose weight, about 25 percent have experienced episodes of binge eating, a key feature of the eating disorder known as bulimia nervosa.

Nurses must understand issues on both ends of

1

the weight management spectrum—obesity and eating disorders—to help patients manage their weight successfully. Both obesity and eating disorders are complex and multidimensional problems that defy simple solutions. Given the lack of success of most current approaches, new approaches to weight management are needed.

This chapter describes why obesity should be viewed as a chronic disease, discusses the relationship between obesity and eating disorders, provides a historical context for understanding obesity and eating disorders, examines trends in the prevalence of obesity and eating disorders, summarizes health concerns associated with body weight changes, and suggests new directions for effective weight management.

VIEWING OBESITY AS A CHRONIC DISEASE

The term obesity carries many negative connotations, including laziness, gluttony, and sloth. So negative are the connotations that the term obesity is often avoided in favor of other less harsh terms, such as overweight. Yet nurses must recognize that obesity is now considered a complex and treatment-resistant chronic disease with multiple causes (National Institutes of Health, 1985). Obese individuals usually do not choose to be obese and have already probably experienced discrimination, prejudice, rejection, and decreased self-esteem. Nurses must counsel obese patients with sympathy and understanding.

Obesity is often viewed as a simple problem of self control—eating too much and exercising too little. Obesity, however, is not one disease but many diseases with complex causes. While the body's energy needs versus the body's energy expenditure are the two primary factors that affect body weight regulation, both of these factors are influenced by complex mechanisms involving genetics; physiol-

ogy; biochemistry; neuroscience; as well as environmental, psychosocial, and cultural factors (Food and Nutrition Board, 1995).

Efforts toward weight loss are usually focused on a fairly brief period of intense treatment followed by far less intense treatment during a maintenance phase. Although losing weight in the first place is, at best, difficult, maintaining the weight loss is even more difficult. Controlled studies show that individuals who complete weight loss programs lose an average of 10 percent of their body weight initially but gain two-thirds of the loss back within a year of discontinuing treatment. They gain almost all of the loss back within five years of discontinuing treatment (National Institutes of Health Technology Assessment Conference, 1992).

Complex biological and environmental forces are often at work causing people to regain lost weight. Thus, successful weight management must focus not only on the short-term weight loss but also, and more importantly, on long-term weight maintenance. Just as management of high blood pressure or type II diabetes requires long-term management and follow-up, so does obesity. Nurses and other health professionals must view obesity not as a social stigma but as a chronic disease that requires life-long vigilance and effort.

INTEGRATING MANAGEMENT OF OBESITY AND EATING DISORDERS

Nurses working in weight management will undoubtedly encounter patients with eating disorders. For susceptible individuals, the onset of an eating disorder often follows a period of restrictive dieting (American Dietetic Association, 1994). A significant proportion of individuals who enroll in weight loss programs exhibit behaviors characteristic of patients with eating disorders (Brownell and Fairburn, 1995).

Weight management covers a broad spectrum ranging from anorexia nervosa to severe obesity, with many areas of overlap in between. Anorexia nervosa is characterized by refusal to maintain a body weight of at least 85 percent of normal weight for height, morbid fear of becoming fat, and a distorted body image. Obesity is characterized by a body weight 20 percent or more above normal weight for height. As different as these two conditions seem, the same basic physiological mechanisms of hunger and satiety apply to both. Similarly, cultural and environmental factors that influence body image and body weight regulation affect individuals with either type of weight problem, though in different ways.

Bulimia nervosa is characterized by recurrent episodes of binge eating coupled with compensatory behavior such self-induced vomiting or misuse of laxatives. Many individuals with bulimia nervosa are normal weight or slightly overweight. Binge eating, a key feature of bulimia nervosa, has been noted in about 25 percent of individuals seeking treatment for weight loss (Brownell and Fairburn, 1995). Obese individuals who exhibit binge eating behavior may be more resistant to treatment than other obese individuals, and vulnerability to obesity is considered a risk factor for bulimia nervosa.

While nurses must recognize overlapping areas in the management of obesity and eating disorders, they must also recognize differences. Dieting is an issue that divides management of the two types of conditions (Brownell and Fairburn, 1995). Dieting is part of the problem for individuals with eating disorders and part of the solution for obese individuals. Obesity research and management have traditionally been described from a medical and physiological perspective, while eating disorders have often been considered a psychological problem. Most individuals cannot fully recover from an eating disorder until the complex issues regarding body image and relationship to oneself and others have been resolved. Treatment of eating disorders, then, has evolved from psychotherapy to also include nutrition therapy. Treatment of obesity has evolved from primarily medical and nutrition therapy to also address psychological and environmental issues.

This course will combine discussion of obesity and eating disorders in areas where they overlap, such as regulation of body weight, health consequences of weight change, and some aspects of nutritional management. Since management approaches have different focuses for obesity versus eating disorders, however, assessment, planning, intervention, and evaluation strategies for these conditions will be described separately.

HISTORICAL PERSPECTIVES

Although isolated cases of obesity have been recognized for thousands of years, obesity as we know it today is a very recent phenomenon. For 95 to 99 percent of our history, humans lived exclusively as hunters and food gatherers (Stuart and Davis, 1972). The change from hunting and gathering to an agricultural society has had important implications for obesity.

The genetic tendency to store excess calories as fat may once have been advantageous. Ironically, as Brown and Konner (1987) have noted, what is now a metabolic problem may once have been a superior survival trait among certain people. That is, some people use less of their food energy stores to produce heat (thermogenesis) and thus have a more efficient energy system. Unfortunately, with easy access to foods, what was originally a boon to the survival of our species may now be a hazard to our health.

Because food shortages were the norm for all

humans under natural conditions, natural selection favored persons who could effectively store calories when food was plentiful to carry them through times when food was scarce. Brown and Konner (1987) have reported that food scarcities would occur at least every two to three years and that fat stores would be depleted in about 75 percent of people.

Women with greater energy reserves had a selective advantage over their leaner counterparts and were better able to withstand the stress of food shortages—not only for themselves but also for their developing fetuses or nursing infants. An early Stone Age statuette, which was viewed as a symbol of fertility, depicts an obese woman with a large abdomen and pendulous breasts (Bray, 1992).

For centuries (and even still today in areas where food is scarce), Nigerian preadolescent girls were housed in a "fattening" room for three months to seven years (depending on the father's wealth) to create a plump, beautiful, and fertile woman (Kocjan and Giannini, 1993).

In ancient times, then, obesity was viewed as a symbol of status and wealth rather than a stigma. Obesity first began to appear more commonly in the English upper classes in the eighteenth and nineteenth centuries, but only since the 1940s has obesity been widely recognized as a health hazard.

Consistent with viewing obesity and overeating as a symbol of status and wealth, wealthy classes from the ancient Greeks and Romans through noblemen of the Middle Ages used to hold great all-day banquets and serve huge amounts of food. It was common for guests to purge themselves by vomiting so they could eat more food.

The Roman Empire institutionalized bulimia in these social rituals by building a vomitarium equipped with fountains, scented water, and flowers adjacent to the dining room where guests could purge themselves in preparation for more eating (Giannini, 1993).

Though the term anorexia nervosa was coined

much later, isolated descriptions of individuals (mostly women) exhibiting its signs and symptoms have appeared in medical literature since ancient times (Slaby and Dwenger, 1993). Prior to the 1900s, descriptions of this wasting condition were often complicated by co-existing medical conditions such as tuberculosis. In the early 1900s, anorexia nervosa was believed to be due to a medical problem with the pituitary gland. In the 1940s emphasis shifted to a psychoanalytical focus, and only recently has emphasis shifted to a neuroendocrine perspective.

Kocjan and Giannini (1993) describe artistic depictions of beautiful women throughout history. Up until the early 1900s, depictions have usually shown realistically proportioned women with protruding stomachs and ample hips. Speaking of changes in the ideal woman since the 1950s, they state "nowhere in history do we see such profound changes in womens' ideal body move so quickly as now." Since the 1980s an unrealistic degree of thinness has come to symbolize success, independence, and attractiveness for women. These unrealistic perceptions combined with the hectic, inactive lifestyles of our times and the abundance of food available have given rise to a greater incidence of obesity and eating disorders than ever before in history.

PREVALENCE OF OBESITY AND EATING DISORDERS

Obesity and eating disorders are primarily Western diseases, occurring predominantly in developed countries where food is plentiful. In Western countries, prevalence of both obesity and eating disorders is at an all-time high and continues to rise.

Based on preliminary data from the Third National Health and Nutrition Examination Survey (NHANES III), 33 percent of Americans over 20

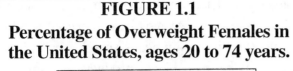

FIGURE 1.1
Percentage of Overweight Females in the United States, ages 20 to 74 years.

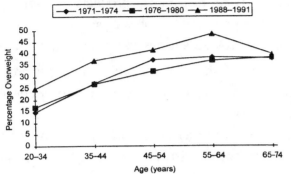

Source: Data are taken from the National Health and Nutrition Examination Survey (NHANES) I (1971–1974), II (1976–1980), and III (1988–1991), conducted by the National Center for Health Statistics. Overweight is defined as >85th percentile for persons 20–29 years, age and gender specific, in NHANES II.

FIGURE 1.2
Percentage of Overweight Males in the United States, ages 20 to 74 years.

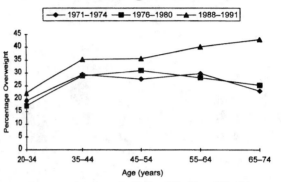

Source: Data are taken from the National Health and Nutrition Examination Survey (NHANES) I (1971–1974), II (1976–1980), and III (1988–1991), conducted by the National Center for Health Statistics. Overweight is defined as >85th percentile for persons 20–29 years, age and gender specific, in NHANES II.

years of age are overweight and 14 percent of Americans are severely overweight (Kuczmarski and colleagues, 1994). About 35 percent of all women, 31 percent of all men, and 25 percent of children and teenagers are considered obese. As shown in *Figures 1.1 and 1.2,* these numbers represent a substantial increase from the Second National Health and Nutrition Examination Survey conducted in the late 1970s, when 27 percent of all women and 24 percent of all men were considered obese (Food and Nutrition Board, 1995).

Today's prevalence of obesity is even higher in subgroups of the population. Individuals with lower levels of education, black women, and Mexican Americans of both sexes have a higher prevalence of obesity. Prevalence of obesity is highest among African Americans, followed by Mexican Americans and European Americans (Williamson, 1995).

For both men and women in the United States, the greatest increase in prevalence of obesity occurs between the ages of 20 to 35 years (Williamson, 1995). The prevalence of obesity increases with age for both men and women and reaches a peak between the 60- to 69-year-old age group for men (42 percent overweight) and in the

50- to 59-year-old age group for women (52 percent overweight).

As shown in *Figure 1.3,* the above numbers are in stark contrast to national health goals for our country. In the landmark report *Healthy People 2000* by the Department of Health and Human Services (1991), the U.S. government set health goals for Americans to reach by the year 2000. According to these goals, no more than 20 percent of adults and no more than 15 percent of adolescents would be overweight by the year 2000. Unfortunately, America is moving farther, rather than closer, to these goals.

Although estimates place the prevalence of eating disorders at somewhere between 2 percent and 10 percent of the U.S. population (Brownell and Fairburn, 1995), eating disorders are not evenly distributed among the population (Hoek, 1995). Young females between the ages of 15 and 24 are most vulnerable to developing eating disorders. Individuals in certain professions, such as professional models or ballet dancers, are also at higher risk. Of those individuals diagnosed with eating disorders in clinical samples, only 5 percent to 10 percent of individuals were males (Hoek, 1995).

Of the eating disorders, bulimia nervosa is far more common than anorexia nervosa. Although the

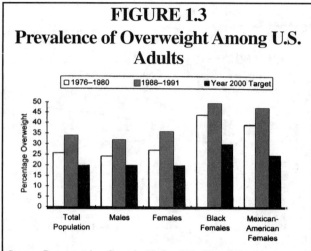

FIGURE 1.3
Prevalence of Overweight Among U.S. Adults

Source: Data are taken from the National Health and Nutrition Examination Surveys (NHANES) II (1976–1980) and III (Phase 1, 1988–1991), conducted by the National Center for Health Statistics, and target goals are taken from *Healthy People 2000* Department of Health and Human Services, 1991.

incidence of anorexia nervosa rose between 1930 and 1970, rates have remained fairly stable since 1970, at about five new cases per 100,000 individuals yearly (Hoek, 1995). Since 1980, however, incidence of bulimia nervosa has increased in epidemic proportions. Some surveys reveal that up to 19 percent of college females report bulimic symptoms (Hoek, 1995). Up to 25 percent of individuals enrolled in weight loss programs report bulimic symptoms (Brownell and Fairburn, 1995).

COSTS OF OBESITY AND EATING DISORDERS

Obesity and eating disorders claim monetary, physiological, and psychological tolls from the individuals they affect. Obesity is a factor in five of the ten leading causes of death in America—coronary heart disease, stroke, high blood pressure, cancer, and diabetes (Surgeon General's Report on Nutrition and Health, 1988).

Since obesity is associated with so many chronic diseases, it is responsible for a large portion of our nation's health care costs. Wolf and Colditz (1994) estimate that direct costs (fees for professional services and hospital care) and indirect costs (value of lost productivity) related to obesity and the associated chronic diseases exceed $68 billion yearly. Since Americans spend over $33 billion yearly on diet-related products and services (U.S. Congress, 1990), obesity and its associated conditions cost Americans over $100 billion yearly.

Although the eating disorders are not as prevalent as obesity, eating disorders are also associated with a variety of health risks. Anorexia nervosa is associated with menstrual and reproductive problems, potentially irreversible osteoporosis and stunting of bone growth, gastrointestinal complications, cardiovascular abnormalities, dehydration, hypokalemia, hypoglycemia, anemia, and neurological complications. Long-term studies reveal a mortality rate of 18 percent in individuals with anorexia nervosa (Goldbloom and Kennedy, 1995). Medical problems associated with bulimia nervosa are similar to those associated with anorexia nervosa, although they are usually less severe (Mitchell, 1995).

In addition to the economic costs, obesity and eating disorders exact a human toll not easily quantified. These conditions are associated with lower self-esteem, depression, discrimination, and social isolation. Gortmaker and colleagues (1993) followed a random national sample of obese adolescents and young adults from 1981 to 1988. Compared to females of normal weight, obese females were significantly less likely to be married, had lower household incomes, and had higher levels of poverty regardless of their baseline socioeconomic status or aptitude scores. Compared to males of normal weight, overweight males were less likely to be married but were similar in other respects.

Unfortunately, discrimination against obese individuals is often ingrained at a very young age. Wadden and Stunkard (1986) reported reactions of children shown pictures of normal weight and obese children:

Children as young as six years describe silhouettes of an obese child as "lazy," "dirty," "stupid," "ugly," "cheats," and "liars." When shown black-and-white drawings of a normal-weight child, an obese child, and children with various handicaps, including mission hands and facial disfigurement, children and adults rated the obese child as the least likable. Not only is this prejudice relatively uniform among blacks and whites and persons from rural and urban settings, it is also, sadly, seen among obese persons themselves.

Studies have also shown that nurses themselves have negative attitudes toward obese individuals. In a study of female university students in a junior nursing class, Stein (1987) noted lower self-concept among obese students compared with nonobese students. Another study evaluated affect neutrality of nurses toward normal-weight and obese patients (Peternelj-Taylor, 1989). In questionnaire analysis, obese patients were evaluated more negatively than patients of normal weight.

NEW WEIGHT MANAGEMENT APPROACHES

Considering the huge economic and personal costs of obesity and eating disorders and the lack of effectiveness of many current programs, new weight management approaches are needed:

- Nurses must recognize that obesity and related eating disorders are chronic diseases that require long-term management. Just as individuals with type II diabetes require long-term follow-up and education, so do individuals with eating disorders or obesity.

- The focus of weight management must become weight maintenance rather than merely weight loss. Too many times patients bounce from one weight loss program or gimmick to another, repeatedly reducing and regaining weight.

- Nurses should help patients set realistic weight goals based on desired health benefits rather than appearance. In many obese individuals, for example, even a 10 percent loss in body weight can produce noticeable improvements in blood pressure, type II diabetes, or blood lipid levels.

- Nurses and other health professionals should help each patient select the best weight management approach based on the patient's needs and preferences. Just as no one blood pressure medication works for every patient, so no one weight management approach works for every person.

- Patients with weight management problems deserve sympathetic and nonjudgmental treatment. Weight management is not simply a matter of self control and willpower; obesity and eating disorders are complex disorders influenced by multiple physiological, psychological, and environmental factors.

This course encompasses management of both obesity and eating disorders because the two so often overlap. The first four chapters of the course are devoted to providing nurses with background information helpful in recognizing and understanding both obesity and eating disorders. Specific aspects of assessment, planning, and intervention for management of obesity and eating disorders are then described in chapters five through twelve. Finally, chapter 13 gives information on weight maintenance and prevention of obesity and eating disorders.

EXAM QUESTIONS

CHAPTER 1
Questions 1–10

1. Nurses should consider obesity to be a problem of
   a. lack of self-control
   b. eating too much
   c. exercising too little
   d. a complex imbalance of energy needs versus energy expenditure

2. Which of the following is true?
   a. The incidence of obesity has decreased slightly in the past five years.
   b. The incidence of eating disorders is now outpacing the incidence of obesity.
   c. Natural selection once favored individuals with increased capacity for thermogenesis.
   d. Obesity was once considered a superior survival trait.

3. In the early 1900s, anorexia nervosa was thought to be due to
   a. sexual abuse
   b. a problem with the pituitary gland
   c. tuberculosis
   d. restrictive toilet training

4. Changes in society's perception of the "ideal woman's" shape have occurred most rapidly during which time period?
   a. the Middle ages
   b. the late 1800s
   c. the early 1900s
   d. the late 1900s

5. About what percent of American adults are overweight?
   a. 14 percent
   b. 20 percent
   c. 33 percent
   d. 50 percent

6. About what percent of American adults are severely overweight?
   a. 14 percent
   b. 20 percent
   c. 33 percent
   d. 50 percent

7. About what percent of females in the United States have serious forms of eating disorders?

   a. 2 percent

   b. 5 percent

   c. 10 percent

   d. 25 percent

8. About what percent of females have mild or variant forms of eating disorders?

   a. 2 percent

   b. 5 percent

   c. 10 percent

   d. 25 percent

9. Among individuals seeking treatment for weight loss, about what percent have engaged in episodes of binge eating?

   a. 2 percent

   b. 5 percent

   c. 10 percent

   d. 25 percent

10. Which of the following should be a new area of focus for weight management programs?

    a. rapid weight loss to reverse chronic disease

    b. weight maintenance over the long-term

    c. willpower and self-control

    d. individualized planning to reach ideal body weight

CHAPTER 2

DEVELOPMENT OF OBESITY AND EATING DISORDERS

CHAPTER OBJECTIVE

After reading this chapter, you will be able to recognize factors that influence body weight regulation and the development of obesity and eating disorders.

LEARNING OBJECTIVES

After studying this chapter, you will be able to

1. Identify factors that affect energy intake and expenditure.

2. Recognize physiological factors influencing the development of obesity and eating disorders.

3. Specify environmental factors influencing the development of obesity and eating disorders.

4. Indicate psychological factors influencing the development of obesity and eating disorders.

INTRODUCTION

The underlying equation governing body weight regulation is *calories in versus calories out*. Patients gain weight if energy intake is chronically greater than energy expenditure. Patients lose weight if energy intake is chronically lower than energy expenditure. Patients maintain weight if energy intake is, on average, about the same as energy expenditure.

While this equation may appear simple, in real-ity a complex web of factors influence both energy intake and energy expenditure, making body weight regulation very complex.

Factors that affect energy intake include

- appetite control
- environmental influences
- availability of food
- diet composition

Factors that affect energy expenditure include

- basal metabolic rate
- level of physical activity
- thermic effect of food (thermogenesis)

Further, an intricate set of mechanisms regulates each of the above factors. Thus, nurses and other health professionals must consider the underlying factors governing body weight in designing appropriate interventions for obesity or eating disorders.

REGULATION OF EATING AND BODY WEIGHT

The regulation of eating and body weight is influenced by numerous physiological, environmental, emotional, social, and cultural influences that all interact (Albright and Stern, 1995). Factors that affect both energy intake and energy expenditure must be considered.

Factors that Affect Energy Intake

Figure 2.1 illustrates some of the factors that influence energy intake. Several physiological factors influence hunger and satiety. Some investigators believe eating behavior is regulated by changes in blood glucose (sugar) levels and glucose availability in the brain—known as the glucostatic hypothesis of feeding (Anderson, 1994). When blood sugar levels fall or when less glucose is being used by the brain, signals are sent to the brain to eat. Glucose availability in the liver also influences glucoreceptors, which provide signals to the brain to initiate eating.

Levels of body fat stores and mobilized free fatty acids may send signals to the brain. Certain regions of the brain are also sensitive to levels of amino acids—the building blocks of proteins—in the body.

The nutritional makeup of the meal itself may influence eating and body weight regulation. Eating high-fat foods and concentrated sweets independently predicts increases in body weight (Albright and Stern, 1995). In rats, eating fat and sugar together causes a greater increase in body weight than eating fat and sugar separately. The combination of sugar and fat increases blood insulin levels and the activity of lipoprotein lipase, an enzyme needed to store fat in body tissues.

Research (Flatt, 1993) suggests that excess fat in the diet promotes obesity more so than carbohydrate or protein. Flatt states that under normal conditions, carbohydrates and proteins are not readily converted to fat. Eating excess calories from carbohydrates or proteins stimulates the breakdown and burning of these fuels, so they are not readily stored as fat in the body. In contrast, excess fat in the diet is readily stored as excess fat in the body, and eating excess fat does not increase the breakdown and burning of fat in the body.

Meal patterns may also influence body weight regulation. In rats fed the same amount of energy daily, those who "nibbled"—ate many small meals daily—gained less weight than rats fed a few large meals daily. Meal patterns may also affect weight regulation in humans (Albright and Stern, 1995).

While many physiological factors affect eating and body weight regulation, many more cultural, social, psychological, and environmental factors mediate or override these responses. Compared to psychosocial and environmental stimuli (especially

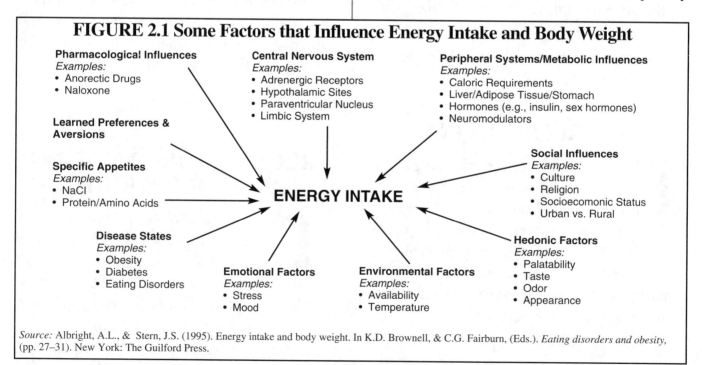

FIGURE 2.1 Some Factors that Influence Energy Intake and Body Weight

Pharmacological Influences
Examples:
• Anorectic Drugs
• Naloxone

Learned Preferences & Aversions

Specific Appetites
Examples:
• NaCl
• Protein/Amino Acids

Disease States
Examples:
• Obesity
• Diabetes
• Eating Disorders

Central Nervous System
Examples:
• Adrenergic Receptors
• Hypothalamic Sites
• Paraventricular Nucleus
• Limbic System

Emotional Factors
Examples:
• Stress
• Mood

Environmental Factors
Examples:
• Availability
• Temperature

Peripheral Systems/Metabolic Influences
Examples:
• Caloric Requirements
• Liver/Adipose Tissue/Stomach
• Hormones (e.g., insulin, sex hormones)
• Neuromodulators

Social Influences
Examples:
• Culture
• Religion
• Socioecomonic Status
• Urban vs. Rural

Hedonic Factors
Examples:
• Palatability
• Taste
• Odor
• Appearance

ENERGY INTAKE

Source: Albright, A.L., & Stern, J.S. (1995). Energy intake and body weight. In K.D. Brownell, & C.G. Fairburn, (Eds.). *Eating disorders and obesity,* (pp. 27–31). New York: The Guilford Press.

those stimuli that have been ingrained and are part of a daily routine), physiological stimuli are usually weaker signals for eating (Smith and Gibbs, 1995).

Factors that Affect Energy Expenditure

While body weight regulation is often equated with food intake, energy expenditure is also a major element of body weight regulation that is often overlooked (Ravussin, 1995). *Figure 2.2* illustrates components of energy expenditure and the factors that influence these components. Basal metabolic rate (BMR, also called resting metabolic rate) is the energy expended by a person who is fasting and at rest in the morning at a comfortable room temperature. BMR accounts for 60 percent to 70 percent of an individual's daily energy expenditure.

Components of body size (such as fat mass and muscle mass), age, and sex explain 80 to 85 percent of the variation in BMR (Ravussin, 1995). Genetic differences probably explain the remaining variability.

A process called thermogenesis accounts for about 10 percent of daily energy expenditure. Thermogenesis is an increase in metabolic rate in response to some sort of stimuli. Food intake, exposure to heat or cold, fear, stress, or administration of certain drugs or hormones trigger thermogenesis. Obese individuals may have less of a thermogenic response to food and other stimuli than lean individuals, perhaps because of the protective fat layers.

Physical activity accounts for 20 percent to 30 percent of total energy expenditure and is the component of total energy expenditure that varies the most from person to person. Not surprisingly, the recent obesity epidemic comes at a time when our society has become more and more sedentary.

Energy expended on physical activity includes energy needed for spontaneous physical activity (small movements) plus voluntary (unrestricted) daily activities and exercise. Although obese indi-

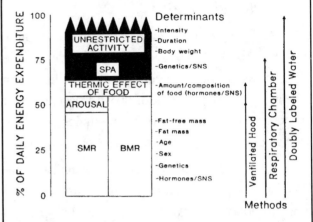

FIGURE 2.2

Components of Daily Energy Expenditure in Humans and Methods of Measurement

Daily energy expenditure can be divided into three major components: the basal metabolic rate (BMR) (sleeping metabolic rate [SMR] + energy cost of arousal), which represents 50% to 70% of daily expenditure; the thermic effect of food, which represents approximately 10% of energy expenditure; and the energy cost of physical activity (spontaneous physical activity [SPA] + unrestricted/voluntary physical activity), which represents 20% to 40% of daily energy expenditure, SNS, sympathetic nervous system.

Source: Ravussin, E. (1995). Energy expenditure and body weight. In K. D. Brownell, & C. G. Fairburn, (Eds.). *Eating disorders and obesity,* (pp. 32–37). New York: The Guilford Press.

viduals tend to move less than lean individuals, it takes more energy to move the greater body mass in obese individuals. Thus, total energy expenditures for physical activity in obese individuals are similar or slightly lower than in lean individuals.

Ravussin (1995) summarized measurements of total energy expenditure over 24 hours in 591 women and 967 men using indirect calorimetry *(Figure 2.3)*. Energy expenditure ranged from 1,251 to 4,381 (average 2,065) calories daily for women and from 1,584 to 4,530 (average 2,462) calories daily for men. Thus, almost all women should lose weight on a calorie intake of less than 1,200 calories daily. Almost all men should lose weight on a calorie intake of less than 1,500 calories daily.

FACTORS INFLUENCING THE DEVELOPMENT OF OBESITY

Genetics and Gender

Obese parents tend to have obese children. About 40 percent of children with one obese parent become obese; when both parents are obese, the risk of obesity rises to about 70 percent (Winick, 1985). Twin studies also provide evidence of the genetic component of obesity.

In twin studies, the weights of identical and fraternal twins have been compared. Other studies have compared the weights of biological parents and their offspring and of adoptive parents and their adopted children. The outcome has usually been that weights tend to be more similar between identical twins than fraternal twins and more similar between biological parents and their offspring than between adopted parents and their adopted children (Bray, 1979; Price and Stunkard, 1989). In a recent study of 4,071 pairs of twins, Stunkard (1986) estimated that about 80 percent of obesity could be explained by genetics.

The Pima Indians living in Arizona also provide researchers with a model of genetic obesity (Ravussin, 1993). About 75 percent of the Pima Indians are obese, indicating that this form of obesity results from a genetically determined efficiency of food use. Mechanisms for the genetic tendency to become obese include a low metabolic rate, decreased ability to waste excess calories as heat (thermogenesis), and a set point for fat cell size. These and other contributors to obesity are discussed in the next sections.

Average body weight differs with race and gender. Overweight increases with age in both sexes. Minority populations have a higher prevalence of obesity than white men and women. Obesity in black women is more common in all age groups than in white women. Although obesity is also

FIGURE 2.3
Energy Expenditure and Body Weight in Males and Females

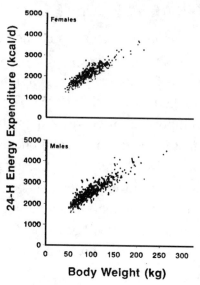

Upper panel: 591 measurements of 24-hour energy expenditure in women with a mean age of 33 ± 12 years (range 18–85 years), body weight of 90 ± 27 kilograms (range 41–320 kilograms), and percentage body fat of 43% ± 9% (range 10%–62%). The mean 24-hour energy expenditure was 2,065 ± 387 kilocalories per day (range 1,251–4,381 kilocalories per day). *Lower panel:* 967 measurements of 24-hour energy expenditure in men with a mean age of 31 ± 10 years (range 18–81 years), body weight of 95 ± 30 kilograms (range 51–266 kilograms), and percentage body fat of 30 ± 11% (range 3%–62%). The mean 24-hour energy expenditure was 2,462 ± 447 kilocalories per day (range 1,584–4,530 kilocalories per day).

Source: Ravussin, E. (1995). Energy expenditure and body weight. In K. D. Brownell, & C. G. Fairburn, (Eds.). *Eating disorders and obesity,* (pp. 32–37). New York: The Guilford Press.

more prevalent among people with lower incomes, the racial differences in obesity rate persist even when controlling for socioeconomic status.

Generally, it is physiologically easier for men to stay thin because their bodies contain more muscle tissue and less fatty tissue than women's bodies. While men may weigh more than women, less of their weight is fat.

Obesity in women is more likely to develop at certain periods of life: the first three years of life, during adolescence, and the third trimester of pregnancy. Women usually gain weight after age 20, during or after pregnancy, and during menopause. Women also start adding fatty tissue during the teenage years because of the release of estrogen. In contrast, men usually lose weight during their teenage years, largely due to the effects of testosterone, which promotes muscle development.

Because men have more muscle tissue than women, they burn calories more quickly than women do. Thus, men need more calories than women to maintain the same weight. Men are almost always taller and heavier than women because of a large skeleton, so they require more energy for activity. Thus, men can lose weight faster than women even though they are eating exactly the same number of calories.

Women's bodies are made up of a much higher percentage of fat. A normal college-aged man's body is made up of about 15 percent fat. A woman's body of the same age, 20 years old, for example, is made up of about 25 percent fat. By the time she reaches 55 years of age, the average proportion of body fat will rise to about 38 percent (Simonson, 1983).

Metabolic Rate

Many obese individuals eat the same amount of food as thin individuals; in fact, many eat less. In contrast, some thin people can eat large amounts of food without gaining much weight (Simonson, 1983). The difference is that the obese individuals may be more fuel-efficient than thinner individuals. Many obese individuals have a lower resting metabolic rate than thinner individuals, so they need fewer calories (Astrup and colleagues, 1996).

Ravussin and Bogardus (1992) documented a large variability in basal metabolic rate among individuals independent of body weight, age, or sex. Some people may genetically have lower energy expenditure, making them at greater risk for obesity (Ravussin, 1993). In fact, prospective studies have shown that a low metabolic rate can predict future obesity in young adults (Ravussin, 1988)

and infants (Roberts, 1988).

Although obese individuals may have lower metabolic rates, their total energy expenditure in 24 hours may actually be higher than that of thinner persons because of the greater energy cost maintaining and carrying around excess weight (Jequier, 1987). This implies that most obese persons must have a greater intake of daily energy than lean persons to maintain body weight and body composition.

Recent starvation, semi-starvation, and rigorous or prolonged dieting can lower basal metabolic rate (Willard, 1991). Suppression of metabolic rate in such situations is the body's attempt to adapt to deprivation and to conserve energy. Thus, dieting can become a contributor to obesity (Simonson, 1983).

Thermogenesis

The role of thermogenesis and its effect on weight and BMR is also of interest. Ingestion of food stimulates the metabolism and produces a demand for energy to meet the multiple activities of digestion, absorption, and transportation of nutrients. Persons who skip meals regularly burn slightly less energy from dietary thermogenesis. Some evidence also indicates that skipping meals may decrease basal metabolic rate (Callaway, 1985).

Many individuals also have the ability to burn off a certain amount of excess calories as heat, a process called adaptive thermogenesis. Obese persons may have decreased adaptive thermogenesis, making them at risk of obesity (Lanzola, 1991).

Diseases of the Endocrine System

Although rare, certain diseases of the endocrine system are associated with obesity (Willard, 1991). Hypercortisolism, polycystic ovaries, hyperinsulinemia, some insulinomas, and hypothyroidism can all promote obesity either through altered metabolism or appetite. Use of inappropriate high doses of insulin in the treatment of diabetes also promotes obesity. Insulin triggers uptake of blood triglycerides into fat cells, favoring storage of excess calories as fat. In fact, the resistance to the action of insulin commonly seen in obesity and type II diabetes may be an adaptive response by the body to prevent additional weight gain (Eckel, 1992).

Adipose Cell Proliferation

Fat is an extremely efficient fuel—that is, this high-energy source has a relatively small volume and thus can be stored in a relatively small space. All forms of life that move use fat or oil as the material in which their energy is stored. This is true not only for fish, animals, and birds, but also for seeds, which are rich in oil and depend on the wind for mobility. In contrast, trees, bushes, and plants, which remain in one place, store energy as carbohydrates.

Although the human body is able to use proteins or carbohydrates as a fuel source, storing large amounts of energy as carbohydrates or proteins would necessitate carrying about ten times the weight of either to gain the same amount of energy as is available from fat. One ounce of fat frees more than twice as much energy as one ounce of carbohydrates or proteins, and it can be stored almost free of water. Each ounce of proteins or carbohydrates is stored with three or four ounces of water.

Our body cells also store fat in a very efficient manner. Each cell, which is about 1/100,000 of an inch in diameter, is enclosed in a thin, flexible membrane that adheres to the membranes of surrounding cells. Fat is stored in connective tissue cells, which have the ability to store tremendous amounts of fat. Any connective tissue cell can become a fat cell merely by filling itself with fat. When it becomes a fat cell, it swells, stretching the cell membrane so that it is no longer ovoid and pointed on each end but round and distended, like a beach ball. It can expand to many times its original size. In addition, the fat in the cell pushes the nucleus out to the edge of the cell. The cell is supplied with a small blood vessel, which acts as a conduit for taking up fats and releasing them back into the bloodstream. Each cell is also supplied with tiny nerve fibers.

Our body is a tremendously efficient energy storage unit—we have millions of connective tissue cells that can easily become fat cells. Thus, our bodies have a nearly unlimited ability to store fat. It is as if, as Gwinup (1970) states, a car's gas tank could swell from a capacity of one gallon to 1,000 gallons, depending on the availability of gasoline.

Recently, much attention has turned to the number and size of fat cells and their influence on weight. A person may have a normal number of fat cells that are swelled with an excess of fat, while another may have too many fat cells. We are all born with our own genetic makeup of fat cells, and some of us are born with more fat cells.

A series of studies first done at Rockefeller University in New York City (Bray, 1985) showed that weight reduction is accompanied by reduction in fat cell size, but not fat cell number. Winick (1985) described what happens when a person with too many fat cells diets down to his or her ideal weight:

> Suppose a person had twice as many fat cells as normal and that each cell contained just the right amount of fat. Such a person would be quite obese, since his or her body would contain twice as much total fat as it should. In order for that individual to achieve normal weight, half of the fat from each cell would have to be burned. Thus, the fat cells would shrink to half their normal size. If now we examined the fatty tissue of this person, who has painfully dieted down to ideal weight, it would appear more abnormal than when he or she was obese.

There would be too many cells, which are now too small as well. The body somehow senses this double abnormality and struggles to rectify the situation by trying to fill those "depleted" fat cells with more fat. For this reason, it is extremely difficult for a person whose obesity is primarily due to too many fat cells to lose weight, and it is even more difficult for that person to maintain the weight loss for a long time.

In contrast, for the person with a normal number of fat cells each containing twice as much fat as it should, weight is easier to lose and weight loss is easier to maintain. As this person loses weight, the fat cells shrink, and when an ideal weight is attained, the fat cells are of normal size. Everything is at the proper levels and thus is much easier to maintain.

How does a person develop an abnormal number of fat cells? Usually the total number of fat cells is reached by early adolescence. Thereafter, fat cells usually increase in size only, not in number. However, fat cells seem to have an upper limit as to how far they can stretch (Willard, 1992). Fat cells in people who are normal weight are about 0.5 μg in diameter. With weight loss, fat cells can decrease to about 0.4 μg. In most types of obesity, fat cells can increase to 0.7 to 1.0 μg, but they rarely exceed 1.5 μg. At this massively obese point, cells have reached their maximum size, and the formation of new fat cells is triggered again. Once more fat cells have been made, they are permanent, making long-term weight loss difficult for severely obese individuals.

Hunger and Satiety Cues

In most people, physiological hunger is carefully regulated by a series of checks and balances controlled by the hypothalamus gland (Blundell, 1990). The hypothalamus senses changes in physical activity and food intake and sends out signals in a very accurate fashion when more food is needed. Interestingly, however, people who are very sedentary may have a faulty check and balance system. Researchers have shown that a low activity level is associated with inappropriately high levels of food intake in both animals and humans (Brownell, 1980).

Though very rare, certain diseases of the hypothalamus, such as Prader-Willi syndrome, can cause voracious appetite and lead to obesity.

Set Point

Obesity is often regarded as a failure of regulation, or lack of balance of intake and expenditure of energy. Biological scientists have found the set point principle useful for describing the systems that regulate such physiologic variables as body temperature and blood pressure. The set point theory of weight is the particular value of a regulated variable at which the system is in balance, or stasis.

According to the set point theory, each person is programmed to have a certain degree of fatness of a body weight at which he or she tends to remain—a set point. Like a thermostat, the set point keeps weight within a relatively narrow range; sometimes it spontaneously jumps, adding a few pounds every five years or so. It is believed that a regulatory mechanism in the brain senses and adjusts both our appetite and our energy use. Thus, when the degree of fat content falls below its programmed amount, and you start to lose weight, you unconsciously desire more food. When you return to your set point, your appetite slackens.

Many obese persons seem to regulate their weight in a normal fashion, and seem to need about the same or slightly more calories for maintaining daily weight as normal-weight persons do.

The basal metabolic rate may also change to suit the circumstances. It automatically slows down to conserve energy and speeds up to burn it, more or less keeping weight stable. Thus, theoretically at least, the set point is a physiological control center that keeps weight at a constant level. For some persons, obesity seems to be regulated. These persons have energy-conserving metabolic adaptations that resist weight change and probably lessen their chances of losing significant amounts of weight or keeping off weight lost through dieting. In order for these people to keep weight off, they must make a lifelong commitment to a daily intake of calories that probably won't satisfy their hunger and that may be less than that consumed by normal-weight persons.

Experts disagree whether a set point for body weight really exists. If it does exist, it may be possible to change a person's set point by adjusting diet and increasing physical activity levels.

Smoking Medications

Some medications can also promote weight gain by increasing appetite or changing metabolism. Such medications include tricyclic antidepressants, phenothiazine, oral contraceptives, and glucocorticoids.

Smoking cigarettes may increase metabolic rate (Perkins, 1989), so when a person stops smoking, weight gain may result. Modest weight gain, however, is still preferable to the unhealthy consequences of smoking. Changes in appetite control may also trigger weight gain after smoking cessation.

Environmental Influences

Going on a series of drastic diets that cause constant weight loss and gain may impair the metabolic process, making it harder to return to a normal weight and stay there. Increased fuel efficiency can also result from being overweight. Persistent overweight, rapid changes in weight, and stringent dieting can slow the body's metabolism down so that a person needs fewer calories daily to maintain

obesity than they did to become obese.

As a person acquires more fatty tissue—which can be maintained at a lower energy cost than muscle tissue—the metabolism slows down so that less energy is expended. The body adjusts, becoming a more efficient machine, that is, it uses less fuel to maintain its needs. When a person stops a very low-calorie diet, the body remains at the lower metabolic rate for weeks or more. With each diet, or each attempt to diet, the energy-savings slowdown of the metabolism is enhanced, making it increasingly difficult to take off pounds.

The family environment greatly influences habitual overeating. When too much food is the norm and where the quantity and the quality of the food are overemphasized by constant conversation about it, it's common for family members to consistently overeat. The types of foods are, of course, also important—it does make a difference if your staple foods are heavy, fried foods, or salads and fresh fruits, with lean meats.

Cultural factors also promote obesity. Eating is a social and recreational activity. The job environment often encourages overeating. Television viewing may also promote obesity. In teenagers, the number of hours spent watching television correlates with prevalence of obesity in an almost linear fashion *(Figure 2.4)*. It is not clear whether excessive television watching causes obesity, or whether the reverse is true.

Obesity is more common among people with lower incomes, particularly among women. Kahn and colleagues (1991) studied 514 black women and 2,770 white women ages 25 to 44 years old over a 10-year interval to determine socioeconomic factors that might predict weight gain. Women most at risk for gaining weight were those without a college education, those who married, and those with very low family incomes. Being a female from a minority population with a low socioeconomic status is considered a triple threat for the

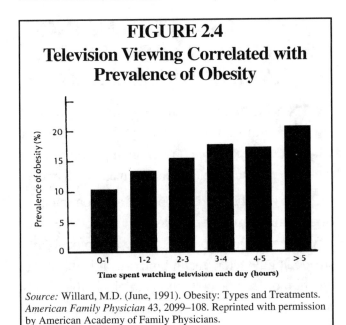

FIGURE 2.4
Television Viewing Correlated with Prevalence of Obesity

Source: Willard, M.D. (June, 1991). Obesity: Types and Treatments. *American Family Physician* 43, 2099–108. Reprinted with permission by American Academy of Family Physicians.

development of obesity (Bowen, 1991).

Sherry and colleagues (1992) studied the effects of socioeconomic status on obesity in children. Contrary to findings in adults, obesity was 50 percent more common in children from higher incomes than from lower incomes, although obesity was the most prevalent growth problem observed in both groups of children.

Psychological Factors

Our society uses food for many reasons besides satisfying hunger. For example, food can be used as a reward for accomplishment, as means of celebrating special occasions, or as a way to express happiness and vitality. Nearly every type of celebration is accompanied by eating and drinking. Despite our culture's strong emphasis on thinness, extravagant overeating is the accepted methods of celebrating any occasion, from weddings and birthdays to Christmas and New Year's Day.

Food can also provide a temporary sense of control over the physical world that surrounds us. In fact, food may at times seem to be the only thing that we can completely control. Food can replace feelings of emptiness, and may compensate for professional or personal failures or for lack of gratification. An individual can fight back against lone-liness and sexual inadequacy with food, or it may help one put aside feelings of depression. In contrast, other people may use food as a target, to get rid of hostility, anger, fear, resentfulness, frustration, or as a release for otherwise unacceptable emotions.

Extra weight can become a barrier between ourselves and our responsibilities. Excess weight may act like a fortress, keeping away unwanted attention or sexuality. Extra weight can be a symbol of power, making a person feel more substantial—someone to be reckoned with and not ignored. Excess weight can also provide a way to avoid competing in a business setting.

Dr. Bruch (1978) is well-known for her work with patients who have eating disorders. She has written that obesity is the consequence of personality defects in which body size becomes the expression of an underlying psychological conflict. According to Bruch, the roots of the problem seem to lie in early life experiences.

Other scientists (Stunkard, 1980; Stuart, 1972) have stated that obesity develops as a result of problems during the "anal" period of childhood development, which is thought to be the point at which a young child seeks to establish his or her independence, while parents try to bring the child's bowel and bladder habits under control. The conflicts during toilet training, when the child attempts to become independent while his parents seek to control him, theoretically lead to the character structure of an adult fixated at or preoccupied with the anal state. Such persons become concerned with orderliness, or compulsiveness, autonomy, and/or defenses against heterosexuality. Psychologists assert that overeating is a compulsive habit in which the person manifests his or her defiance of those who would control his eating while at the same time protecting him or herself from heterosexual experiences by virtue of the invulnerability or unattractiveness of excess weight.

Some people love to eat not because they need to satisfy a deep-seated emotional need but because they can't deny themselves anything they really want, including the pleasure of eating. Some were trained from early on to be "good children," which meant eating heartily and cleaning every scrap from their plates. In adulthood, many overeaters still feel that limiting their intake of food is a betrayal of their parents and family traditions, even if their parents are no longer around to remind them to eat everything on their plates (Stuart, 1972).

Bruch theorized that one of the mechanisms by which parents inadvertently induce their children to become obese is through inappropriate use of food in response to varying emotional stress signals by the child, and conversely a failure to respond with food when the child becomes hungry. Because of this, food can become an inappropriate response to almost any strong emotion; thus, we may learn highly inappropriate responses and develop inappropriate food habits. Eating disturbances are often the result of pathogenic interaction between the individual and key figures in his or her environment.

In the late 1960s, Schachter (1971) and colleagues developed the hypothesis that people of normal weight eat in response to internal physiological cues, especially hunger, whereas obese people eat because of external cues in their immediate environment. Thus, instead of feeling hungry and then eating as a response, obese persons eat in response to the time of day, the sight and nearness and accessibility of food, or the sight of other people eating. To test this theory, Schachter devised a study in which he changes the clocks in the study room to reflect a later time, closer to dinner time. The obese persons in the study ate twice as many snack crackers when they thought it was 6 P.M. than when they thought it was 5:20 P.M. Normal-weight persons acted in a very different way: they ate less, as if they were "saving" themselves for dinner.

FACTORS INFLUENCING THE DEVELOPMENT OF EATING DISORDERS

Eating disorders most commonly occur among adolescent or young women in developed societies. Often a period of dieting precedes the development of an eating disorder.

Like obesity, the development and continuation of an eating disorder depends on multiple genetic, physiological, environmental, psychological, and sociocultural factors that all interact. It is this combination of factors, not one factor alone, that determines whether or not an individual will develop an eating disorder.

Cooper (1995) has proposed three stages in the development and maintenance of an eating disorder *(Figure 2.5)*. Stage one represents the period of time from conception to the development of a behavioral precursor of the eating disorder, which is often dieting. During this stage, many predisposing factors can occur, which increase the likelihood of the individual developing an eating disorder.

Stage two represents the period of time between the development of behavioral precursors of the eating disorder and onset of the frank disorder. During this stage certain precipitating factors can increase the likelihood of the individual developing a full-blown eating disorder.

Stage three represents the period of time between the onset of the full-blown disorder and the time when the disorder is well established and considered chronic. Certain maintaining and protective factors intervene during this stage to determine if the eating disorder will be temporary and transient or chronic and established.

Psychological Factors

Certain psychological factors may predispose patients to develop eating disorders (Cooper, 1995). Low self-esteem and perfectionism are traits frequently reported in individuals with both

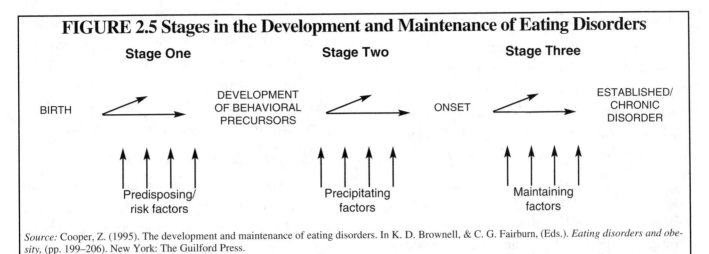

FIGURE 2.5 Stages in the Development and Maintenance of Eating Disorders

Source: Cooper, Z. (1995). The development and maintenance of eating disorders. In K. D. Brownell, & C. G. Fairburn, (Eds.). *Eating disorders and obesity,* (pp. 199–206). New York: The Guilford Press.

anorexia nervosa and bulimia nervosa. Excessive compliance has also been reported in individuals with anorexia nervosa. These traits may predispose individuals who then diet to develop behavioral precursors to eating disorders.

Individuals with eating disorders more frequently have histories of an affective disorder compared with individuals who do not have eating disorders (Cooper, 1995). Prevalence rates of major depression in patients with both anorexia nervosa and bulimia nervosa range from 25 percent to 80 percent. High levels of anxiety symptoms have been documented in patients with both types of eating disorders. Obsessive-compulsive personality disorder has been frequently noted in individuals with anorexia nervosa, while borderline personality disorder has been frequently noted in individuals with bulimia nervosa.

Although researchers have noted certain traits or affective disorders in patients presenting with eating disorders, more research is needed to determine whether the traits and affective disorders existed before the eating disorder developed or whether they are a result of the disorder.

Physical Risk Factors

Individuals with an eating disorder have often been obese before the development of the disorder. Cooper (1995) reports that 7 to 20 percent of patients with anorexia nervosa and 18 to 40 percent

of patients with bulimia nervosa were obese prior to developing the eating disorder. Cooper hypothesizes that the obesity leads people to diet, and dieting is a predisposing factor for eating disorders.

Some evidence suggests that alterations in the neurochemical system of the brain and neuroendocrine processes may predispose certain individuals to developing eating disorders. Studies of individuals with anorexia nervosa, bulimia, and common eating problems such as food cravings, seasonal appetite disturbances, and stress-related eating suggest altered levels of the amines and neuropeptides in cerebrospinal fluid (Leibowitz, 1995). Others suggest that feeding difficulties early in infancy may also be a predisposing factor to eating disorders (Cooper, 1995).

Family History

Relatives of individuals with eating disorders are three times as likely to develop an eating disorder themselves as are relatives of individuals without eating disorders (Cooper, 1995). This increased risk may be due to both genetic and environmental factors. Genetic factors may operate through other predisposing factors, such as increased risk for obesity or increased rates of other affective disorders such as depression or mood disorder.

A family history of substance abuse, such as alcohol abuse, is also a risk factor for developing eating disorders, particularly bulimia.

Environmental Factors

Family environment influences the development of an eating disorder. Certain family patterns seem to be more common in patients with eating disorders, but it is unclear whether these patterns predispose individuals to develop eating disorders or whether they are a result of the eating disorder (Cooper, 1995).

In self-reports of family interactions (Vandereycken, 1995), patients with bulimia nervosa often describe their family as "conflicted, badly organized, noncohesive, and lacking in nurturance and caring." In contrast, patients with anorexia nervosa describe their families as "stable, nonconflictual, cohesive, and with no lack of nurturance."

In observer reports of family interactions in these patients, families of anorexic patients were described as more rigid, having less clear interpersonal boundaries, and avoiding disagreements between parents and children. Observer reports of families of patients with bulimia were more similar to self-reports. Bulimic patients were seen as being "angrily submissive to rather hostile and neglectful parents."

Stressful life events can also trigger the development of anorexia nervosa and bulimia nervosa. Individuals with eating disorders have higher rates of childhood sexual abuse than individuals without eating disorders (Palmer, 1995). Considering the age at which eating disorders commonly develop, patients who have suffered childhood sexual abuse may be more sensitive to emerging issues of sexuality and self-concept. It is unclear whether such stressful life events themselves predispose an individual to develop an eating disorder, or whether they work through other predisposing factors, such as psychiatric problems or patterns of family interaction.

Social and Cultural Factors

In developed countries, society puts enormous pressure on individuals—especially women—to be thin. The constant bombardment of media messages from newspapers, magazines, television, and billboards sets unrealistic standards for many individuals. Thinness is equated with success, self-worth, status, control, and competency; while obesity is associated with laziness, self-indulgence, and lack of willpower (Wilfley and Rodin, 1995).

These pressures cause many women and some men to be dissatisfied with their body shape and to diet, which may predispose them to development of an eating disorder. In a review of the psychological consequences of dieting, Polivy (1996) noted that starvation and rigid self-imposed dieting resulted in preoccupation with food and eating and binging when food was available.

Young women are still developing their identify and are particularly sensitive to issues of shape and weight. The fact that eating disorders occur predominately in developed countries that place such an emphasis on thinness underscores the significance of sociocultural factors in the development of eating disorders.

The next chapter reviews the medical implications of obesity and eating disorders.

EXAM QUESTIONS

CHAPTER 2
Questions 11–17

11. Which of the following factors affect energy expenditure?

    a. thermic effect of food

    b. appetite control

    c. availability of food

    d. food cues

12. Basal metabolic rate accounts for about what percent of total daily energy expenditure?

    a. 20 to 30 percent

    b. 40 to 50 percent

    c. 60 to 70 percent

    d. 80 to 90 percent

13. Physical activity accounts for what percent of total daily energy expenditure?

    a. 0 to 10 percent

    b. 20 to 30 percent

    c. 40 to 50 percent

    d. 60 to 70 percent

14. Which of the following is true?

    a. About 40 percent of children with one obese parent become obese.

    b. About 40 percent of children with two obese parents become obese.

    c. Almost 100 percent of children with two obese parents become obese.

    d. Parental obesity does not affect the child's chances of becoming obese.

15. Which of the following is true?

    a. Obesity is less common among adults with lower incomes compared to adults with higher incomes.

    b. Obesity is more common in children of higher income families than in children of lower income families.

    c. Obesity is less common in children of higher income families than in children of lower income families.

    b. Incidence of obesity and socioeconomic status of children and adults are not related.

16. Parents sometimes inadvertently encourage obesity in their children by

    a. withholding food

    b. disciplining too harshly

    c. using food inappropriately in response to varying emotional signals in the child

    d. offering too great a variety of foods at mealtimes

17. Which of the following is a predisposing factor that increases the likelihood of developing an eating disorder in susceptible individuals?

    a. depression

    b. restrictive dieting

    c. euphoria

    d. excessive exercising

CHAPTER 3

MEDICAL COMPLICATIONS OF OBESITY AND EATING DISORDERS

CHAPTER OBJECTIVE

After reading this chapter, you will be able to identify health implications of obesity, weight loss, weight regain, and eating disorders.

LEARNING OBJECTIVES

After studying this chapter, you will be able to

1. Identify the relationship between body weight and mortality.

2. Specify obesity-related risk factors for cardiovascular disease.

3. Recognize medical complications of obesity.

4. Specify the effects of weight cycling.

5. Identify medical risks of anorexia nervosa and bulimia nervosa.

INTRODUCTION

Obesity is a risk factor in five of the ten leading causes of death in America. Obesity also exacerbates several other health conditions. Losing only 10 to 15 percent of body weight triggers significant improvement in conditions like high blood-lipid levels, high blood pressure, and non-insulin-dependent diabetes. However, weight loss followed by weight regain may also carry risks.

Eating disorders lead to multiple medical complications, some of which can be fatal. Eating disorders are associated with bone and muscle wasting, fluid and electrolyte imbalances, menstrual and endocrine irregularities, irritation or even rupture of the gastrointestinal tract, and dental complications.

This chapter will review the relationship of body weight to mortality rate, the health consequences of obesity, the health benefits of weight loss, the effects of the "yo-yo" syndrome of weight loss and regain, and the medical consequences of anorexia nervosa and bulimia nervosa.

BODY WEIGHT AND MORTALITY

Life insurance statistics clearly show that weight extremes are linked to increased mortality. Data from the Build Study of 1979 (American Society of Actuaries and Association of Life Insurance Medical Directors of America, 1980) show that the lowest mortality rates are in those individuals slightly under established weight for height in life insurance tables. Weights above or below this norm are associated with increased mortality. Thus, the relationship between overall mortality and body mass index is J-shaped (Van Itallie, 1992). This J-shaped curve applies to mortality from cardiovascular diseases, cancer, diabetes, hypertension, gallbladder diseases, and osteoporosis (Bray, 1985).

Others have described the effects of gross obesity on life expectancy. In one study, 200 morbidly-obese men whose average weight was 143.5 kg (315.7 lb) were interviewed when they were admitted to a weight-control program. These men were followed for an average of five years. Their ages ranged from 23 to 70 years, with a mean of 42.7 years.

The mortality of this group was higher at every age when compared with the mortality expected for males in the general public. The excess mortality for men aged 25 to 34 was an astonishing 1,200 percent. For those 35 to 54 years of age, the excess mortality declined to 550 percent, and for men 55 to 64 years of age, the mortality was only twice that of the normal-weight men in the general population. Excess mortality associated with obesity is greatly increased in younger persons, and not surprisingly, excess mortality is substantially higher in grossly obese persons.

Recent studies have shown that the weight range associated with lowest mortality increases with age in both men and women (National Institutes of Health Consensus Conference, 1985), indicating that excess weight later in life is not as harmful as excess weight earlier in life. In fact, Mattila and colleagues (1986) report that survival among people 65 years of age or older is greater in individuals with a higher body mass index.

Other studies document the negative effects of excess weight in younger persons. In several studies, men who became overweight early in life had more cardiovascular problems later. For example, Abraham and colleagues (1971) related the changes in weight status between childhood and adult life to the incidence of hypertension, cardiovascular, and renal disease in 715 males. Childhood weight was determined from school weights recorded when these men were 9 to 13 years of age. They were then reweighed at an aver-

age age of 48 years. The highest incidence of hypertension and cardiovascular-renal disease was recorded in men with the lowest childhood weight who had become overweight as adults.

In a similar study, Must (1992) related weight status in adolescence to morbidity and mortality later in life. Men and women who initially participated in the Harvard Growth Study of 1922–1935 were studied. For subjects who had died, cause of death was determined from death certificates. The average age of subjects at follow-up was 73 years. About 52 percent of living subjects who were overweight as adolescents were still overweight at follow-up. Male subjects who were overweight as adolescents had twice the death rate as lean adolescents, regardless of adult weight. Death rate from coronary heart disease, atherosclerotic cerebrovascular disease, stroke and colon cancer was higher in these subjects. In contrast, women who were overweight as adolescents did not have higher overall or disease-specific death rates compared to women who were lean as adolescents. However, overweight women had a 1.6 higher incidence of arthritis.

Insurance studies and data from the ongoing Framingham study have shown that losing excess pounds may prolong life. In both men and women who successfully lost and maintained a lower body weight during their lifetimes, mortality rates were reduced to within normal limits for sex and age. In the Framingham study, reducing body weight by 10 percent decreased incidence of coronary artery disease by 20 percent (Kannel, 1986).

The Framingham Study

The Framingham study is perhaps one of the longest and best-publicized surveys of the effects of nutrition and weight on health, particularly cardiovascular health. More than 5,000 residents of Framingham, Massachusetts, have been followed for nearly three decades to find epidemiological clues to the development of cardiovascular disease and other illnesses.

After following the population for 26 years, 870 men and 688 women in the Framingham study had died (Hubert and colleagues, 1983). Relative weight at the time a person entered the study was found to be an independent predictor of cardiovascular disease, particularly in women. Researchers were able to predict the incidence of coronary artery disease and death rate from coronary artery disease. The likelihood of developing heart failure in men was predicted from the initial degree of obesity. The predictive power of obesity was independent of age, cholesterol level, systolic blood pressure, cigarette smoking, or glucose intolerance.

Researchers concluded that obesity is an important and long-term predictor of cardiovascular disease, particularly in younger persons. In women, only age and blood pressure levels were more powerful predictors. In men over 30 years of age in the study, the lowest mortality occurred at a relative weight of 100 percent to 109 percent of ideal body weight for both smokers and nonsmokers. Based on results of the Framingham study, there would be 25 fewer cases of coronary disease and 35 percent fewer cases of congestive heart failure and stroke if everyone were at their optimal weight.

American Cancer Society Study

The American Cancer Society published the results of a prospective study of more than 750,000 persons between 1959 and 1972 (Simonson, 1983). In this study, relative death rates among subgroups of people whose weights deviated above or below average established body weights were compared with the death rates for groups with average body weights (90 to 109 percent of ideal).

Subjects were divided into two groups—smokers and nonsmokers. A smoker of normal body weight had an increased mortality rate comparable to that of a moderately obese nonsmoker. There was no increase in death rate until body mass reached 25 kg/m^2. Body mass index (BMI) is the weight in kg divided by the height in meters squared. Excess weight also had a profound effect on death from diabetes and gallbladder disease.

In this study, the incidence of cancer could be correlated with weight status. As the BMI increased, there was an increase in cancer deaths, although the effect was much slighter than other causes of death. Obese males had significantly higher rates of prostate and colon-rectal cancer. For women, obesity could be correlated with a much higher incidence of cancer of the gallbladder, breasts, cervix, endometrium, uterus, and ovary.

The Gothenberg Study

Two Scandinavian studies—the Gothenberg study and the Norwegian study—also provided interesting data about the effects of obesity on health. The Gothenberg study (Lapidus and colleagues, 1984), conducted with 450,000 residents of southwest Sweden, is similar to the Framingham study. This study contributed new information on the health consequences of moderate obesity.

In men, the BMI and ratio of waist-to-hip circumference were positively correlated in individuals who eventually developed strokes. Men with the highest waist-to-hip ratio and the highest BMI had a 20.8 percent risk for developing strokes compared to a 5.6 risk for men with the lowest BMI and lowest waist-to-hip ratio. Surprisingly, the greatest risk of cardiovascular disease was reported in men with the highest waist-to-hip ratio and the lowest BMI.

Among the 14,462 women 38 to 60 years old in the study, death rates from heart attack, stroke, and all causes were related to the waist-to-hip fat ratio. Women with the highest ratios had an 8.2 times more risk of heart attack than women with the lowest ratios.

The Norwegian Study

The Norwegian study (Waaler, 1983) used a

different technique to study a majority of the Norwegian population between 1963 and 1975. A nationwide x-ray screening program provided height and weight measurements for a large proportion of the people in Norway. A total of 1,717,000 men and women aged 15 to 90 were followed during the 12-year study.

Minimal mortality rates for men and women occurred at a BMI of 23. There was a steep increase in death rate when the BMI was lower than 23. Between a BMI of 23 and 27 there was a curvilinear increase in excess mortality. Among obese persons, the principal causes of death were cerebrovascular disease, cardiovascular disease, diabetes mellitus, and cancer of the colon. Researchers concluded that excess mortality could have been reduced by 15 percent if all subjects had been closer to their ideal weights.

The Nurses' Health Study

Data on risk factors for coronary heart disease in women are sparse. The Nurses' Health Study (Manson, 1990) examined the influence of current obesity, relative weight at the age of 18, and inter-

vening weight gain on subsequent risk of fatal and nonfatal coronary heart disease. This large-scale prospective study included 115,886 healthy females who were also registered nurses. Follow-up was over an eight-year period.

Subjects were divided into five weight categories based on BMI. After eight years, obesity was shown to be a strong risk factor for fatal and nonfatal coronary heart disease *(Figure 3.1)*. Subjects in the highest weight category had 3.3 times the risk for heart disease as subjects in the lowest weight category. In the heaviest women, 70 percent of coronary heart disease events were attributable to obesity. Even mild to moderate overweight was associated with increased risk of coronary heart disease.

Current body weight was more predictive of coronary heart disease than weight at age 18. Further, weight gain between age 18 and current age substantially increased coronary risk. Nurses who gained 10 to 19.9 kg (22 to 44 pounds) during adulthood had a 60 percent greater risk of developing coronary heart disease than nurses who gained

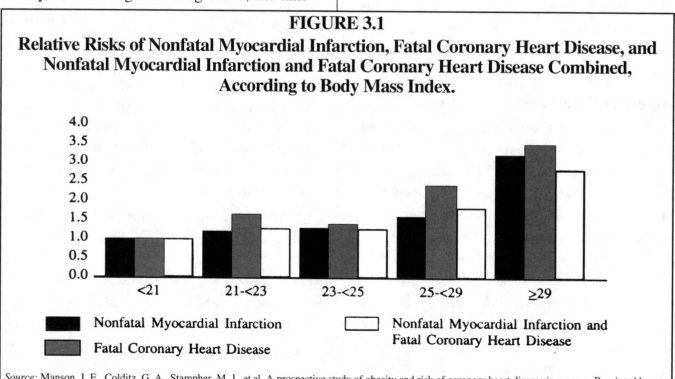

FIGURE 3.1

Relative Risks of Nonfatal Myocardial Infarction, Fatal Coronary Heart Disease, and Nonfatal Myocardial Infarction and Fatal Coronary Heart Disease Combined, According to Body Mass Index.

Source: Manson, J. E., Colditz, G. A., Stampher, M. J., et al. A prospective study of obesity and risk of coronary heart disease in women. Reprinted by permission of *The New England Journal of Medicine,* 322, 882–889, 1990.

less than 3 kg (6 pounds). Nurses who gained 20 to 34.9 kg (44 to 77 pounds) had over a 200 percent greater risk of developing coronary heart disease.

The Swedish Obesity Study

Recent results of the ongoing Swedish Obesity Study (SOS) provide evidence of the long-term benefits of weight loss (Sjostrom and colleagues, 1994; Nabro and colleagues, 1994). The SOS consists of a nationwide sample of 10,000 severely obese individuals 37 to 59 years of age. Initially, BMI values averaged 37.5 for men and 40.6 for women in the study. The study examined the health of participants and compared the long-term effects of weight loss through surgical means versus conventional means. A total of 856 individuals were selected for surgical intervention and were matched with 856 controls.

Healthy obese subjects with the highest BMI levels had the highest risk of all-cause mortality. Other factors such as fat distribution, fasting blood insulin levels, and smoking also independently predicted mortality. Of the 442 individuals who underwent surgical intervention and were followed for two years, weight losses averaged 28 kg compared to less than 1 kg in matched controls. Obesity-related risk factors improved significantly in the surgical group, as did current health, mood, and other obesity-related problems.

HEALTH RISKS OF OBESITY

Cardiovascular Disease

Atherosclerosis develops early in life and progresses as we age. Fatty materials, or lipids, carried in the blood as cholesterol are deposited in the lining of arteries and form rough plaques that slowly increase in size. With time, the plaque builds up and gradually reduces the opening in the artery through which blood flows. The artery can become completely blocked, cutting off the blood supply to the area it serves. If this happens to be a portion of the brain, a stroke occurs. If it is a coronary artery, a heart attack occurs.

Besides being an independent risk factor for cardiovascular disease (CVD), obesity aggravates other risk factors such as hyperlipidemia, hypertension, and diabetes. Wolf and Colditz (1994) estimate that the direct costs of obesity-related cardiovascular disease exceed $29.4 billion. As following sections describe, CVD risk profiles usually improve with weight loss.

Several factors beyond our control influence the risk of developing atherosclerosis and subsequent cardiovascular diseases. Males have a higher risk of cardiovascular disease than females, and risk increases with age for both males and females. Black individuals have a higher risk than white individuals. Individuals with a strong family history of cardiovascular disease are also at greater risk of developing the disease.

In addition to the factors we cannot control, other factors that we can control influence the risk of atherosclerosis and cardiovascular disease. Five major modifiable risk factors for atherosclerosis include high blood cholesterol levels (hyperlipidemia), high blood pressure (hypertension), cigarette smoking, diabetes, and obesity. Although the type A personality pattern characterized by aggressiveness, ambition, impatience, and a chronic sense of time urgency used to also be considered a risk factor, many recent studies have cast doubt on this theory. In fact, individuals tending toward a type A personality may recover from heart attack better than more relaxed individuals tending toward a type B personality (Case, 1985).

Hyperlipidemia

Risk for heart disease increases with increasing serum cholesterol levels in a curvilinear fashion, with risk sharply rising with total cholesterol levels above 240 mg/dl. Desirable blood cholesterol levels are less than 200 mg/dl, with levels between 200 and 239 mg/dl considered borderline-high and levels of 240 mg/dl or more considered high. Cholesterol contributes to atherosclerosis and CVD by clogging blood vessels and blocking blood flow.

Cholesterol is manufactured in the body and is also present in food. Serum levels are determined by the availability of cholesterol from these two sources. Most of the endogenous cholesterol in our bodies is manufactured by the liver, then transported to other organs as needed. Many of the hormones produced by the adrenal gland are made from cholesterol. The insulation around nerve sheaths in the brain is mostly cholesterol. The gallbladder uses cholesterol to produce bile. Thus, cholesterol is essential for life and only becomes a health hazard when it occurs in excess amounts.

The body regulates the amount of cholesterol in the blood, producing less in the body if more is provided by the diet. However, this protective mechanism can be overwhelmed when people consume large amounts of cholesterol and saturated fats, found in animal foods such as meat and dairy products.

Cholesterol is transported in the blood attached to proteins, forming lipoproteins. Most cholesterol is carried by low-density lipoproteins, or LDLs. High levels of LDL cholesterol in the blood greatly increase risk for atherosclerosis. Desirable LDL cholesterol levels are less than 130 mg/dl, with levels of 130 to 159 mg/dl considered borderline, and levels of 160 mg/dl or more considered high. Levels of LDL cholesterol almost always correlate with high levels of total cholesterol.

A small amount of cholesterol in the blood is carried by another protein called high-density lipoprotein, or HDL. A higher level of HDL cholesterol in the blood is desirable because it protects against atherosclerosis. Desirable levels of HDL cholesterol in the blood are 35 mg/dl or greater.

Hyperlipidemia, or elevated blood lipid levels,

is more prevalent in obese individuals than in lean individuals. Many obese individuals have elevated blood triglyceride levels, reduced HDL cholesterol levels, and an elevated ratio of LDL to HDL cholesterol (Food and Nutrition Board, 1995). Such a pattern of hyperlipidemia substantially increases risk for cardiovascular disease.

Thirty-two percent of overweight men have high blood cholesterol levels, compared to 22 percent of lean men (National Heart, Lung and Blood Institute, 1993). The figures are similar for women. Thirty-eight percent of overweight women compared to 25 percent of lean women have high blood cholesterol levels. Data from the Framingham study and the Second National Health and Nutrition Examination Survey confirm that mean serum cholesterol levels increase with increasing body weight.

While obesity increases risk for hyperlipidemia, weight loss decreases it. Weight loss has been shown to correlate with decreases in serum total cholesterol levels (Osterman and colleagues, 1992). Weight losses of 5 to 10 percent will increase blood HDL levels (Wood and colleagues, 1988). In a six-week study using a low-fat, low-calorie diet, weight losses of 5 to 6 percent of initial body weight were associated with 16 percent decreases in total cholesterol levels and 12 percent decreases in LDL cholesterol levels (Seim and Holtmeier, 1992).

Hypertension

Hypertension, or high blood pressure, is defined as a systolic blood pressure of 140 mm Hg or more and/or a diastolic blood pressure of 90 mm Hg or more. More Americans visit their physician for hypertension than for any other disorder, and antihypertensive medications are the most frequently prescribed drugs in America (Kanders and Blackburn, 1992).

The prevalence of high blood pressure in overweight individuals is more than twice that of lean individuals (National Heart, Lung and Blood Institute, 1993). Fifty-five percent of obese men have high blood pressure compared to 27 percent of lean men. Fifty-two percent of obese women have high blood pressure compared to 19 percent of lean women. Similar to high blood cholesterol levels, the mean level of both systolic and diastolic blood pressure increases in linear fashion with increasing body weight (National Institutes of Health, 1993).

High blood pressure accelerates atherosclerosis. A person with a systolic blood pressure greater than 160 mm Hg or a diastolic blood pressure greater than 95 mm Hg has a five-fold increase in risk of coronary heart disease compared to persons with normal blood pressure. Hypertension poses the greatest risk in persons older than 45 years of age and is a strong predictor of stroke.

The association between obesity and hypertension has long been recognized. When weight is lost, blood pressure usually drops. For example, hypertension nearly vanished among people who had great caloric deprivation during World War II. Bray (1985) noted that 50 to 80 percent of persons who lose weight also have a reduction in blood pressure. Studies have shown that this drop occurs even when the sodium content of the diet was kept constant.

Schotte and Stunkard (1990) reported that weight losses of 10.4 kg in obese individuals who were hypertensive and not receiving their antihypertensive medications still reduced systolic blood pressure by 15.8 mm Hg and diastolic blood pressure by 13.6 mm Hg. In the Framingham study, weight losses of 15 percent were associated with a 10 percent reduction in systolic blood pressure (Kannel and colleagues, 1967).

Many other studies have also documented that weight loss reduces blood pressure, including one study that reported a 1 mm Hg reduction in both systolic and diastolic blood pressure for every kilo-gram of weight loss in young, obese women with hypertension (McMahon and colleagues, 1985). The National Institutes of Health (1993) recommends weight loss as a key goal for obese individuals with hypertension.

Other dietary factors that may influence blood pressure include potassium, calcium, magnesium and dietary fat intake (National Institutes of Health, 1993). High potassium intake may protect against developing high blood pressure. Calcium deficiency may make a person more at risk of developing high blood pressure. Preliminary studies suggest that low dietary magnesium intake may also increase risk for high blood pressure, though these studies need to be confirmed. A certain type of fat, the omega-3 fatty acids found in rich concentrations in fatty fish such as salmon, mackerel and haddock, may also help lower blood pressure.

Diabetes

Diabetes, one of the most serious yet relatively common problems in modern times, results from a deficiency of insulin—a hormone produced by the pancreas. There are two main forms of diabetes. Type I diabetes, also called insulin-dependent diabetes mellitus (IDDM) usually occurs in childhood and is characterized by a complete inability to manufacture insulin in the body. Type II diabetes, also called non-insulin-dependent diabetes (NIDDM) usually develops later in life and is characterized by varying ability to make insulin and resistance to the action of insulin in the body.

Type I diabetes is due to an absolute lack of insulin. The mechanisms within the pancreas that produce insulin are damaged and can no longer produce insulin. This severe type of diabetes must be treated quickly with insulin, which the patient must take for life. Dietary changes cannot prevent this type of diabetes, but dietary intake must be controlled and carefully matched with insulin taken.

Type II diabetes also results from a deficiency

of insulin. In this form of diabetes, however, the pancreas may produce some insulin, but not enough to keep up with the body's needs or become resistant to the action of insulin. Type II diabetes usually develops later in life and tends to run in families. Some groups, such as Ashkenazie Jews, African Americans, and American Indians, are at greater risk of developing diabetes. Dietary modification can have a powerful impact on this type of diabetes.

Diabetes is the third most frequent cause of death in the United States (Perri, 1992). Obesity is a strong risk factor for type II diabetes. About 80 percent of people with diabetes have type II diabetes. Of these individuals, 80 to 90 percent are obese. In fact, obesity is probably the single most important factor in the development of type II diabetes, and weight loss is the most important treatment long-term goal.

About 60 percent of individuals with severe obesity eventually develop type II diabetes (Grundy, 1990). The longer the duration of obesity, the greater the risk of developing type II diabetes (Everhart, 1992).

Individuals with type II diabetes show improved glucose control within days of starting a weight loss program (Food and Nutrition Board, 1995). This immediate effect is probably due to lowered energy intake. As body weight is lost, sensitivity to the action of insulin increases, further improving blood glucose control. For many individuals with type II diabetes, weight losses of 10 to 15 percent of body weight allows patients to discontinue taking insulin or oral antidiabetic agents. Weight loss can even normalize blood glucose control in some individuals.

Diabetes is also associated with high blood pressure. The resistance to insulin that commonly occurs in type II diabetes may explain the link between diabetes and high blood pressure. Insulin resistance may also explain the link between dia-

betes and hyperlipidemia and cardiovascular disease (DeFronzo, 1991). The mechanisms by which insulin resistance could trigger high blood pressure are not clearly understood but could involve sodium retention in the body, overactivity of the sympathetic nervous system, disturbances in ion transport across membranes, or proliferations of vascular smooth muscle cells.

High insulin levels in the body and insulin resistance promote hyperlipidemia by causing the body to manufacture more very low-density lipoproteins, leading to higher levels of triglycerides and low-density lipoproteins in the blood. High levels of insulin are also known to promote atherosclerosis independent of insulin's effects on blood fat levels.

Thus, obesity and overweight powerfully affect the development and course of diabetes.

Cancer

The risk of cancer increases with increasing body weight. In a large-scale study of 750,000 subjects conducted by the American Cancer Society (Lew, 1979), risk of cancer was increased in both obese men and women, particularly in those over 40 percent of ideal weight, compared to their lean counterparts. In obese men, cancer of the colon, rectum, prostate, pancreas, and stomach were increased. In obese women, cancer of the endometrium, breast, gallbladder, cervix, and ovary were increased.

The death rate from cancer for men who were 40 percent or more overweight was one-third higher than for men of average weight. The death rate for cancer among women who were 40 percent or more overweight was 55 percent higher than for women of average weight.

Obesity increases risk of endometrial cancer during the premenopausal as well as postmenopausal years. Women who weigh more than 30 percent of ideal weight have twice the risk of this cancer, while women who weigh more than 40 percent of ideal weight have four times the risk. In contrast, the risk for breast cancer increases with obesity only after menopause.

Obese people have increased levels of prolactin, androgens, estrogens, and cortisol. Several studies have singled out estrogen as having a role in development of cancers of the reproductive system, such as endometrial, cervical, breast, and ovarian cancer. Adipose tissue is the major site of estrogen formation.

Breast cancer is the most common cancer that affects American women and is a leading cause of death in the United States. In fact, American women experience a far greater incidence of breast cancer than women in other countries. Scientists who have tried to find a common link to this type of cancer have come up with one possibility: a diet high in fat. The more fat a population consumes, no matter how highly developed or primitive the country is, the higher the incidence of breast cancer. Obese women also have a slightly higher incidence of uterine cancer than lean women. This is particularly true for women who have been obese since childhood (Lew, 1979).

Colon cancer is very common in the U.S., and its incidence is increasing. A recent study suggests that overweight during middle-age or young adulthood increases risk of developing colon cancer (Lee, 1992). The best correlation of cancer of the colon is with a diet high in fat. Unlike breast cancer, men are just as likely to develop colon cancer as women. Theories about development of colon cancer suggest that a high-fat diet changes the normal bacterial flora of the large intestine. Bacteria transform the fat into other products, some of which may act as carcinogens.

Diets low in fiber contribute to colon cancer. Fiber is the portion of the carbohydrate within food that is indigestible and not absorbed by the body. Fiber is present in the outer layer of cereal grains, known as bran, and in the skin and fleshy portions

of fruits and vegetables. Dietary fiber also attracts water to it. As fiber passes through the gastrointestinal tract, it will soften the stool, speeding passage through the large intestine and decreasing the time carcinogens come in contact with the intestinal wall.

Other Problems

Obesity increases risk or exacerbates several other problems and diseases. Obesity is a primary contributor to sleep apnea—very brief periods of time during sleep when an individual stops breathing (Young and colleagues, 1993). Sleep apnea can cause an individual to feel sleepy and less alert during the day. It is also a risk factor for premature death.

Obesity is a risk factor for osteoarthritis of weight-bearing joints such as the knee, hip, and back. Weight loss significantly improves symptoms and management of osteoarthritis (deGennes, 1993).

The work of breathing is increased when considerable additional weight is carried on the chest wall. In addition, excessive fatty tissue also increases the complexity of getting oxygen to all the tissues of the body. As a result of reduced oxygenation, obese persons have lower tolerance levels for exercise and may even have difficulty in normal breathing, particularly with a respiratory infection.

The Pickwickian syndrome, which was named after Dickens' character Joe, a fat boy in the *Pickwick Papers,* is marked by hypoventilation, somnolence, and obesity. Losing weight is essential for treatment of the Pickwickian syndrome.

Thousands of people undergo treatment for gallstones each years. Gallbladder disease and digestive disease in general are more common in obese persons (Kato, 1992). The incidence of digestive diseases is 40 percent above the normal level in persons who are 15 to 35 percent overweight and nearly 150 percent above normal in those who are 65 percent or more overweight. The

American Cancer Society study also showed that overweight persons are more likely than normal-weight persons to die from digestive diseases.

Hirsutism and menstrual irregularities are much more common among obese women, and can often be improved by weight loss.

Overweight can also cause problems during pregnancy. The risk of toxemia and delivery problems can be reduced if weight is controlled, preferably before pregnancy occurs. Obese men may be troubled by infertility.

Obesity may be an important risk factor in the development of diverticular disease (Schauer, 1992). Obesity, excessive weight gain in young adulthood, and high blood pressure are also risk factors for the development of gout (Roubenoff, 1991).

Body Fat Distribution

The type of obesity present also influences health risks. Upper body obesity (excess fat more in the trunk and abdominal areas) is more dangerous than lower body obesity (excess fat more in the buttock and hip areas). A waist-to-hip ratio of above 0.85 for women and 0.95 for men is associated with hypertension, hyperlipidemia, diabetes, and increased coronary heart disease mortality (Despres, 1990). Women with central obesity are also at greater risk of breast cancer than women with lower body obesity (Schapiru, 1990).

Fat deposits around the area of major body organs may pose a greater strain on the body than fat in extremities. Also, fat deposits in the trunk and abdominal areas are more metabolically active than fat deposits in the lower body, promoting insulin resistance and its associated problems of high blood pressure, diabetes, abnormal blood lipid levels, and cardiovascular disease (Bjorntorp, 1991).

HEALTH BENEFITS OF WEIGHT LOSS

Even modest weight losses of about 10 to 15 percent of body weight (20 to 30 pounds for someone weighing 200 pounds, for example) improve health and decrease medical problems in 90 percent of obese patients (Blackburn, 1987). Modest weight losses improve heart function, blood pressure, blood sugar control, sleep disorders, and blood lipid profiles. Such weight losses also decrease the need for medication, hospitalizations, and postoperative complications (Robison, 1993).

In a review of the effects of weight loss in obese patients, Goldstein (1992) noted significant health improvements in patients with type II diabetes, high blood pressure, high blood cholesterol levels, and cardiovascular disease when they lost about 10 percent of body weight. Such modest losses also appeared to increase longevity in obese individuals.

Weight loss decreases the incidence and severity of both hypertension and type II diabetes. Recent studies have even suggested weight loss may prevent the onset of these diseases for some people (National Institutes of Health, 1992). Weight loss also reduces or eliminates the need for medication in some people with diabetes or high blood pressure.

Cardiovascular risk directly decreases with weight loss. Data from the Framingham study suggest that a 10 percent decrease in body weight corresponds to a 20 percent decrease in risk of developing coronary artery disease (Ashley, 1974). Modest weight losses also decrease cardiovascular risk in women, even when they still remain obese (Tremblay, 1992).

Besides physical benefits, weight loss in very obese persons has been associated with better self-esteem, improved functional status, reduced work absenteeism, less pain, and greater social interaction.

HEALTH RISKS OF WEIGHT LOSS

Although the health benefits of weight loss are well documented, weight loss can also have some negative effects (National Institutes of Health, 1992). Persons on very strict weight loss diets often report fatigue, hair loss, and dizziness. Weight loss in persons who are only slightly overweight leads to greater loss of lean body mass (muscle tissue) than in severely overweight individuals. Dieting may also increase the risk of developing an eating disorder.

The health effects of repeated weight loss and regain (weight cycling) are unclear (Robison, 1993). Some studies suggest that weight cycling may change the way the body handles energy.

A study by Stein and colleagues (1986) showed that wrestlers who repeatedly lost and regained weight had slower metabolisms than those who did not. Decreases in metabolic rate were associated with weight loss and regain in obese women (Jequier, 1990). Studies with rats also suggest that weight cycling increases the efficiency of feeding, that is, more weight is gained on less food. Thus, a person who loses a large amount of weight and then rapidly regains it theoretically may have a lowered metabolic rate, making weight loss more difficult and increasing the likelihood of regaining weight during the next dieting attempt.

However, not all studies of weight cycling support these conclusions. Robison (1993) has shown that the lowered metabolism with dieting to be only a temporary effect, and one that does not occur with diets containing at least 1,200 calories. Some studies also suggest that weight cycling may increase death rate, particularly from heart disease (Lissner, 1991), whereas other studies fail to sup-

port such findings (Jeffrey, 1992). Repeated failure to maintain weight loss may also contribute to the poor self-esteem experienced by many obese persons. Though still unclear, the possible negative effects of weight loss and regain deserve further study.

HEALTH RISKS OF EATING DISORDERS

Since eating disorders represent a complex interplay of physical and emotional factors, health consequences are both psychological and physical. In addition to feelings of guilt, isolation, depression, and lack of control, eating disorders are associated with bone and muscle wasting, fluid and electrolyte imbalances, menstrual and endocrine irregularities, irritation or even rupture in various sites in the gastrointestinal system, and dental complications.

Most of these medical risks resolve quickly with normalization of feeding patterns and weight restoration. Some medical complications of eating disorders—such as bone loss—may affect the individual for the rest of his or her life. Though less common, some complications of eating disorders can be fatal. In fact, the death rate for patients suffering from anorexia nervosa is around 18 percent (Goldbloom and Kennedy, 1995).

Many of the medical complications seen in eating disorders are a result of starvation and the body's adaptive response to it (deZwaan and Mitchell, 1993). In earlier military studies where healthy men were subjected to starvation conditions to simulate prisoner-of-war camps, the men soon developed many features common in patients with anorexia nervosa (Keys and colleagues, 1950). These men felt tired and depressed and became obsessed over food. They ate meals slowly and with strange rituals during the starvation phase. When they were re-fed, they exhibited behaviors of binge eating for months afterwards.

Although there is no typical patient and all patients must be thoroughly assessed, health consequences of bulimia nervosa are usually less serious than the consequences of anorexia nervosa. While patients with anorexia nervosa are, by definition, seriously underweight, most patients with bulimia nervosa have a near-normal body weight or are slightly overweight. Health effects of disturbed eating behaviors are summarized in *Table 3.1* and discussed in the next two sections. Since overlap occurs in health aspects of anorexia nervosa and bulimia nervosa, nurses and clinicians must carefully evaluate each patient.

Medical Complications of Anorexia Nervosa

Perhaps no other psychiatric disorder has as many medical complications as does anorexia nervosa (Goldbloom and Kennedy, 1995). Medical complications of this disorder can affect all body systems, including endocrine, bone, gastrointestinal, cardiovascular, renal, blood, skin, and neurological complications.

In females, lack of menstrual periods is a diagnostic criteria, although menstruation stops before significant weight loss occurs in about one-third of patients (Mickley, 1994). Anorexia nervosa is associated with disturbed hormonal patterns. In females, reversion to or maintenance of prepubertal hormone secretory patterns frequently occurs. In males, altered hormonal patterns are manifested as sexual disinterest or dysfunction. Infants of women with active anorexia during pregnancy have lower-than-average birth weights and lower scores on standard neonatal tests.

Studies suggest individuals with anorexia nervosa have a reduced rate of bone formation and an increased rate of bone resorption, possibly due to low estrogen levels and elevated cortisol levels. These changes are potentially irreversible and can lead to stunting of growth and osteoporosis (Goldbloom and Kennedy, 1995). Bone complications are one of the most serious effects of anorexia nervosa.

Anorexia nervosa also alters gastrointestinal functions. Food takes longer to travel through the

TABLE 3.1 Medical Complications of Eating Disorders

Abnormal Eating and Weight Regulating Behaviors	Consequences
Binge eating	Mechanical irritation and dilatation of the stomach "Overnutrition"
Starvation, chaotic eating pattern	Excessive weight loss → metabolic and endocrine adaptation Malnutrition → nutritional deficits
Self-induced vomiting	Mechanical irritation → injuries of the upper GI tract, injuries of the mediastinum Fluid and electrolyte abnormalities → organ system dysfunctions
Laxative abuse	Mechanical irritation → injuries of the lower GI tract Fluid and electrolyte abnormalities → organ system dysfunctions Addiction
Diuretic abuse	Fluid and electrolyte abnormalities → organ system dysfunctions Addiction
Diet pills	Addiction
Ipecac syrup	Vomiting, toxicity

Source: deZwaan, M., & Mitchell, J. E. (1993). Medical complications of anorexia nervosa and bulimia nervosa. In A. S. Kaplan & P. E. Garfinkel, (Eds.). *Medical issues and the eating disorders: the interface.* (pp. 1–16). New York: Brunnel/Mazel Publishers.

gut, causing constipation, stomach bloating, and abdominal pain. Both the starvation state itself and the abuse of laxatives contribute to these gastrointestinal complications. Patients who use stimulant laxatives (such as Ex-lax and Correctol) for long periods of time can permanently damage nerve function in the colon. These laxatives work for the bowel, making it unable to function properly on its own after prolonged use. In rare instances, acute dilation, bleeding, or perforation of the stomach can occur, particularly during rapid refeeding or uncontrolled overeating.

The muscle wasting that occurs from starvation during anorexia nervosa affects not only visible muscles like the arms and legs, but also hidden muscles like the heart. The heart muscle becomes smaller and weaker, leading to cardiac abnormalities. Low heart rate (with rates as low as 30 beats per minute), low blood pressure, and decreased circulation to the extremities can occur. Often the toes and fingers can appear bluish to purplish, especially in the cold. Mitral valve prolapse can also occur.

Any individual with an eating disorder who uses syrup of ipecac to induce vomiting should be carefully evaluated. The emetine in this product has a long half-life and can build up in the body to dangerously high levels even if used only two or three times weekly (Mickley, 1994). Emetine is a muscle poison and can cause sudden heart failure.

Patients with anorexia nervosa, especially those who purge by vomiting, laxative, or diuretic abuse can become dehydrated and develop electrolyte abnormalities. Chronic dehydration and low potassium levels in the blood can cause irreversible damage to the kidneys. Anorexia is also associated with mild forms of anemia, yellowish discoloration of the skin, the appearance of fine, downy body hair (lanugo), and disturbances in both central and peripheral neurological function.

Death rate in patients with anorexia nervosa is about 18 percent (Goldbloom and Kennedy, 1995)—unusually high compared with death rates for other psychiatric disorders. Cardiac complications and changes in electrolyte and fluid balance account for much of the mortality associated with anorexia nervosa.

Medical Complications of Bulimia Nervosa

Although patients with bulimia nervosa exhibit behavior extremes—consuming enormous amounts of food and then purging—medical complications of bulimia nervosa are usually much less serious than complications of anorexia nervosa (Mitchell, 1995). The most common symptoms patients complain of include fatigue, lethargy, bloating, nausea, constipation, abdominal, tooth sensitivity, and irregular menstrual periods.

Tell-tale signs of bulimia include enlargement of the salivary glands (most often the parotid glands), which manifests itself as puffy cheek; calluses or irritation on the back of the hand (so-called Russell's sign), which arise from repeatedly using the hand to stimulate the gag reflex; and dental enamel erosion in the mouth, which occurs in most patients who have been vomiting for four years or longer. Swelling and edema is sometimes found in individuals who abuse laxatives and diuretics. About 20 percent of individuals with bulimia nervosa also abuse alcohol or drugs (Mickley, 1994).

Several gastrointestinal complications are common in patients with bulimia. The salivary glands can become swollen, giving the cheeks a puffy appearance. The esophagus can become inflamed from stomach acid during vomiting. Gastric reflux can cause heartburn. The stomach empties slowly, can dilate, and even tear. Gastric rupture is one of the most common causes of fatality in patients with bulimia (Mitchell, 1995). Patients with bulimia also frequently experience constipation, especially when abusing laxatives that work for the bowel.

Patients with bulimia frequently have irregular

or absent menses. Pregnancy in individuals with bulimia poses new medical problems since it increases fetal risks.

Patients with bulimia who purge through vomiting or laxative or diuretic abuse lose fluid and often become dehydrated. About 50 percent of patients with bulimia have electrolyte abnormalities, most often metabolic alkalosis because of potassium loss in the urine and chloride loss from vomiting (Mitchell, 1995). Some patients who abuse laxatives can also develop acidosis from loss of bicarbonate-rich fluid in the stool.

As in patients with anorexia nervosa, any history of abuse of syrup of ipecac merits careful evaluation, since the emetine is stored in muscle—including the heart—and can cause problems with contraction.

The next chapter defines degrees of obesity and types of eating disorders and provides guidelines for diagnosis.

EXAM QUESTIONS

CHAPTER 3
Questions 18–26

18. The lowest mortality rates are associated with body weights

    a. 20 percent under recommended weights

    b. slightly under recommended weights

    c. slightly over recommended weights

    d. 20 percent over recommended weights

19. The relationship between overall mortality and body mass index is

    a. straight-lined

    b. U-shaped

    c. J-shaped

    d. exponential

20. Desirable serum total cholesterol levels for adults are

    a. below 200 mg/dl

    b. 200 to 220 mg/dl

    c. 220 to 240 mg/dl

    d. above 240 mg/dl

21. Elevation of which type of cholesterol in the body is most associated with increased risk of cardiovascular disease?

    a. very low-density lipoprotein cholesterol

    b. low-density lipoprotein cholesterol

    c. intermediate-density lipoprotein cholesterol

    d. high-density lipoprotein cholesterol

22. About what percentage of people with non-insulin-dependent diabetes are also obese?

    a. 20 to 30 percent

    b. 40 to 50 percent

    c. 60 to 70 percent

    d. 80 to 90 percent

23. Which of the following statements regarding obese individuals is true?

    a. Weight losses of five percent of body weight can significantly improve health.

    b. Weight losses of 10 to 15 percent of body weight can significantly improve health.

    c. Significant improvements in health status are seen only with weight losses of over 25 percent of body weight.

    d. Once obesity-related health problems occur, they cannot be reversed.

24. Which of the following is a possible effect of weight cycling?

    a. improved health status

    b. increased lean body mass

    c. lowered body metabolism

    d. reduced cardiovascular disease risk

25. Which medical complication of eating disorders may be irreversible?

    a. nutritional deficiencies

    b. bone losses

    c. menstrual irregularities

    d. electrolyte imbalances

26. The death rate for patients suffering from anorexia nervosa is about

    a. 5 percent

    b. 12 percent

    c. 18 percent

    d. 25 percent

CHAPTER 4

DEFINING OBESITY
AND EATING DISORDERS

CHAPTER OBJECTIVE

After studying this chapter, you will be able to differentiate between normal weight, overweight, obesity, and eating disorders.

LEARNING OBJECTIVES

After reading this chapter, you will be able to

1. Discriminate between the term overweight and the term obese.

2. Indicate meaning and uses of various body weight indices.

3. Identify signs of anorexia nervosa.

4. Identify signs of bulimia nervosa.

5. Recognize signs of atypical eating disorders.

INTRODUCTION

Health professionals often use the terms overweight, obese, anorexic, or bulimic loosely. However, for accurate diagnosis and effective management, each of these terms must be clearly defined. This chapter will differentiate between overweight, obesity, and severe obesity based on weight-for-height tables and body mass index. The importance of body fat distribution will also be discussed. Finally, diagnostic criteria for anorexia nervosa, bulimia nervosa, atypical eating disorders, and binge-eating disorder will be given.

OVERWEIGHT VERSUS OBESE

The terms obesity and overweight are often used interchangeably. Referring to a patient as "overweight" sounds less negative and harsh compared to using the term "obese." The two terms, however, have different meanings. While obesity refers to an excess of body fat, overweight refers to weighing more than normal for height and build, but not necessarily due to excess body fat.

For example, a well-muscled football player who is 6′4″ tall could easily weigh 240 pounds and be in excellent health. Yet, according to height and weight charts he would be 40 pounds overweight. Although he is overweight, he is not overfat or obese, just well muscled. Since most of us are not professional football players, most Americans who are overweight are also obese.

The term overweight is frequently used to describe someone who weighs up to 20 percent above recommended weight according to a weight-for-height table.

DEFINING OBESITY

All of us have some body fat. A certain amount of body fat is necessary for storing energy and supporting and cushioning organs. The term obesity, however, refers to an abnormally large percentage of body fat that impairs health (National Institutes of Health Consensus Conference, 1985). But how much fat is normal and how much is unhealthy?

Generally a total body fat content of more than 25 percent for men and more than 30 percent for women is considered to represent obesity (National Institute of Diabetes and Digestive and Kidney Diseases, 1993).

Body fat can be measured directly using underwater weighing, measuring skinfold thicknesses at several body sites, scanning by dual-energy X-ray absorptiometry (DEXA), bioelectrical impedance analysis (sending a very small electric current through the body), or total body electrical conductivity (TOBEC, which is based on an interaction between the body and a varying magnetic field). Because many of these methods for assessing body fat content require complex equipment and trained personnel, their use is not practical in most clinical settings.

Body fat can also be estimated indirectly. The two most common and easily determined techniques for indirectly assessing obesity include weight-for-height tables and body mass index (BMI).

Weight-for-Height Tables

Weight-for-height tables were developed in the 1940s and 1950s by the life insurance industry as a guide to evaluate life insurance applicants. Insurance industry standards were established because overweight people were poor insurance risks and were required to pay higher premiums, if they were offered coverage at all.

Although life insurance tables have become widely used, their utility in defining obesity has been questioned. One problem is that people with the lowest mortality rates tend to weigh less than the weight ranges given. Another problem is that insurance policy holders represent a select subset of the general population: they are largely white, middle-class adult males; and individuals with chronic disease or acute illnesses are often not included in life insurance statistics because they do not apply for insurance or are rejected. Also, body weights are often self-reported and inaccurate.

Despite these limitations, weight-for-height tables based on life insurance data are widely used because of their simplicity. The 1959 Metropolitan Life Desirable Weight Table (Society of Actuaries, 1959) has been used for years and continues to be the table of choice for many clinicians. As shown

TABLE 4.1 Desirable Weights for Men and Women Age 25 and Over

MEN					WOMEN				
HEIGHT			**FRAME**		**HEIGHT**			**FRAME**	
Feet	Inches	Small	Medium	Large	Feet	Inches	Small	Medium	Large
5	2	112–120	118–129	126–141	4	10	92–98	96–107	104–119
5	3	115–123	121–133	129–144	4	11	94–101	98–110	106–122
5	4	118–126	124–136	132–148	5	0	96–104	101–113	109–125
5	5	121–129	127–139	135–152	5	1	99–107	104–116	112–128
5	6	124–133	130–143	138–156	5	2	102–110	107–119	115–131
5	7	128–137	134–147	142–161	5	3	105–113	110–122	118–134
5	8	132–141	138–152	147–166	5	4	108–116	113–126	121–138
5	9	136–145	142–156	151–170	5	5	111–119	116–130	125–142
5	10	140–150	146–160	155–174	5	6	114–123	120–135	129–146
5	11	144–154	150–165	159–179	5	7	118–127	124–139	133–150
6	0	148–158	154–170	164–184	5	8	122–131	128–143	137–154
6	1	152–162	158–175	168–189	5	9	126–135	132–147	141–158
6	2	156–167	162–180	173–194	5	10	130–140	136–151	145–163
6	3	160–171	167–185	178–199	5	11	134–144	140–155	149–168
6	4	164–175	172–190	182–204	6	0	138–148	144–159	153–173

Source: Data adapted from the Statistical Bulletin, Metropolitan Life Insurance Company, New York. Derived primarily from data of the *1959 Build and Blood Pressure Study,* Society of Actuaries.

TABLE 4.2 1983 Metropolitan Height-Weight Tables

HEIGHT (WOMEN)		FRAME*			HEIGHT (MEN)		FRAME*		
Feet	Inches	Small	Medium	Large	Feet	Inches	Small	Medium	Large
4	10	102–111	109–121	118–131	5	2	128–134	131–141	138–150
4	11	103–113	111–123	120–134	5	3	130–136	133–143	140–153
5	0	104–115	113–126	122–137	5	4	132–138	135–145	142–156
5	1	106–118	115–129	125–140	5	5	134–140	137–148	144–160
5	2	108–121	118–132	128–143	5	6	136–142	139–151	146–164
5	3	111–124	121–135	131–147	5	7	138–145	142–154	149–168
5	4	114–127	124–138	134–151	5	8	140–148	145–157	152–172
5	5	117–130	127–141	137–155	5	9	142–151	148–160	155–176
5	6	120–133	130–144	140–159	5	10	144–154	151–163	158–180
5	7	123–136	133–147	143–163	5	11	146–157	154–166	161–184
5	8	126–139	136–150	146–167	6	0	149–160	157–170	164–188
5	9	129–142	139–153	149–170	6	1	152–164	160–174	168–192
5	10	132–145	142–156	152–173	6	2	155–168	164–178	172–197
5	11	135–148	145–159	155–176	6	3	168–172	167–182	176–202
6	0	138–151	148–162	158–179	6	4	162–176	171–187	181–207

* Weights at ages 25 to 50, based on lowest mortality. Height includes 1-inch heels. Weight for women includes 3 lbs. for indoor clothing. Weight for men includes 5 lbs. for indoor clothing.

Source: Metropolitan Life Insurance Company, 1983.

in *Table 4.1,* the 1959 Metropolitan Life Insurance Table gives desirable weight ranges for men and women age 25 years and over according to frame size. A desirable weight range for a medium-frame woman measuring 5 feet, 5 inches tall, for example, would be 104 to 116 pounds.

Most weight-for-height tables are set up to include variations depending on body frame or relative size of bones. This is also a controversial area, and some scientists believe that frame types were created simply by dividing the weight distribution of all the life insurance data into thirds and labeling those thirds "small," "medium," or "large." Even the American Medical Association has pointed out the difficulties of determining frame size. For others, however, frame size gives one more variable to help determine appropriate weight.

Simonson (1983) suggested the following two methods for estimating frame type:

1. Measure your height to the nearest quarter of an inch. Have someone else measure the circumference of your shoulders with a tape measure. Add the two figures. If the total of the two measurements is less than 99 inches, you have a small frame. If the total is 99.1 to 106.0 inches, you have a medium frame. If the total is more than 106 inches, you have a large frame.

2. Measure the circumference of the wrist on your dominant hand. For women, a wrist measurement less than 6 inches indicates a small frame, 6 to 6½ inches indicates a medium frame, and over 6½ inches indicates a large frame. For men a wrist measurement less than 6 inches indicates a small frame, 6 to 7 inches indicates a medium frame, and more than 7 inches indicates a large frame.

In March 1983, the Metropolitan Life Insurance Company issued its new and adjusted weight ranges for men and women based on data for 4.2 million persons over 22 years. The 1979 Build Study (Society of Actuaries and Association of Life Insurance Medical Directors of America, 1980) showed that the gap between average population body weights and weights associated with lowest mortality had narrowed. Thus, the 1983 tables allow higher body weights than those reported in 1959 (*see Table 4.2*). The 1983 tables also avoid the terms "ideal" or "desirable" body weight.

TABLE 4.3 Suggested Weights for Adults, Federal Government, 1990

Weight (pounds)[b]

Height[a]	19-34 Years Old	35 Years Old and Over
5'0"	97–128	108–138
5'1"	101–132	111–143
5'2"	104–137	115–148
5'3"	107–141	119–152
5'4"	111–146	122–157
5'5"	114–150	126–162
5'6"	118–155	130–167
5'7"	121–160	134–172
5'8"	125–164	138–178
5'9"	129–169	142–183
5'10"	132–174	146–188
5'11"	136–179	151–194
6'0"	140–184	155–199
6'1"	144–189	159–205
6'2"	148–195	164–210
6'3"	152–200	168–216
6'4"	156–205	173–222
6'5"	160–211	177–228
6'6"	164–216	182–234

NOTE: The higher weights in the ranges generally apply to men, who tend to have more muscle and bone; the lower weights more often apply to women, who have less muscle and bone.

[a]Without shoes.

[b]Without clothes.

Source: U.S. Departments of Agriculture and Health and Human Services, *1990 Dietary Guidelines for Americans,* 1990.

Many clinicians have been critical of these higher weight ranges and prefer to continue using the 1959 tables (VanItallie and Simopoulos, 1994). They believe that clinicians should emphasize preventing obesity and beginning treatment at lesser degrees of obesity.

In 1990 the federal government used a weight-for-height table in its Dietary Guidelines for Americans (U.S. Departments of Agriculture and Health and Human Services). As shown in *Table 4.3*, the suggested weights in this table increase for individuals 35 years of age and older. This table has been criticized (VanItallie and Simopoulos, 1994) both for not being based on science and for implying that it is acceptable to gain weight with increasing age.

The 1995 version of the Dietary Guidelines for Americans (U.S. Departments of Agriculture and Health and Human Services) includes a simplified weight-for-height graph showing healthy weight ranges, moderate overweight ranges, and severe overweight ranges for men and women combined *(Figure 4.1)*. The higher body weights apply to people with more muscle and bone mass, such as many men.

No one body weight is right for everyone, and body weight varies not only with body fat content but also with body muscle and bone content. While weight-for-height charts are simple and easy to use, they give only general guidance regarding healthy weights and degree of obesity.

Relative Weight

The term "relative weight" expresses a patient's weight in pounds as a percentage of desirable body weight as defined in weight-for-height tables. Relative weight is calculated by dividing current weight in pounds by the midpoint of the desirable weight range.

Consider, for example, a woman who is five feet eight inches tall and weighs 165 pounds. Using the 1983 Metropolitan Life Insurance Tables from the previous section, the midpoint of the medium-frame weight range for this height is 143 pounds.

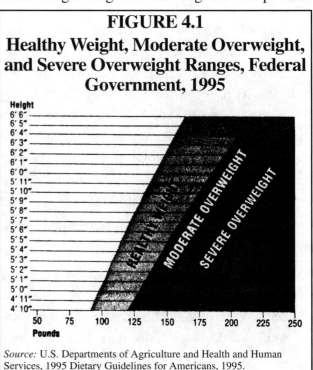

FIGURE 4.1
Healthy Weight, Moderate Overweight, and Severe Overweight Ranges, Federal Government, 1995

Source: U.S. Departments of Agriculture and Health and Human Services, 1995 Dietary Guidelines for Americans, 1995.

CHAPTER 4

DEFINING OBESITY
AND EATING DISORDERS

CHAPTER OBJECTIVE

After studying this chapter, you will be able to differentiate between normal weight, overweight, obesity, and eating disorders.

LEARNING OBJECTIVES

After reading this chapter, you will be able to

1. Discriminate between the term overweight and the term obese.

2. Indicate meaning and uses of various body weight indices.

3. Identify signs of anorexia nervosa.

4. Identify signs of bulimia nervosa.

5. Recognize signs of atypical eating disorders.

INTRODUCTION

Health professionals often use the terms overweight, obese, anorexic, or bulimic loosely. However, for accurate diagnosis and effective management, each of these terms must be clearly defined. This chapter will differentiate between overweight, obesity, and severe obesity based on weight-for-height tables and body mass index. The importance of body fat distribution will also be discussed. Finally, diagnostic criteria for anorexia nervosa, bulimia nervosa, atypical eating disorders, and binge-eating disorder will be given.

OVERWEIGHT VERSUS OBESE

The terms obesity and overweight are often used interchangeably. Referring to a patient as "overweight" sounds less negative and harsh compared to using the term "obese." The two terms, however, have different meanings. While obesity refers to an excess of body fat, overweight refers to weighing more than normal for height and build, but not necessarily due to excess body fat.

For example, a well-muscled football player who is 6'4" tall could easily weigh 240 pounds and be in excellent health. Yet, according to height and weight charts he would be 40 pounds overweight. Although he is overweight, he is not overfat or obese, just well muscled. Since most of us are not professional football players, most Americans who are overweight are also obese.

The term overweight is frequently used to describe someone who weighs up to 20 percent above recommended weight according to a weight-for-height table.

DEFINING OBESITY

All of us have some body fat. A certain amount of body fat is necessary for storing energy and supporting and cushioning organs. The term obesity, however, refers to an abnormally large percentage of body fat that impairs health (National Institutes of Health Consensus Conference, 1985). But how much fat is normal and how much is unhealthy?

Generally a total body fat content of more than 25 percent for men and more than 30 percent for women is considered to represent obesity (National Institute of Diabetes and Digestive and Kidney Diseases, 1993).

Body fat can be measured directly using underwater weighing, measuring skinfold thicknesses at several body sites, scanning by dual-energy X-ray absorptiometry (DEXA), bioelectrical impedance analysis (sending a very small electric current through the body), or total body electrical conductivity (TOBEC, which is based on an interaction between the body and a varying magnetic field). Because many of these methods for assessing body fat content require complex equipment and trained personnel, their use is not practical in most clinical settings.

Body fat can also be estimated indirectly. The two most common and easily determined techniques for indirectly assessing obesity include weight-for-height tables and body mass index (BMI).

Weight-for-Height Tables

Weight-for-height tables were developed in the 1940s and 1950s by the life insurance industry as a guide to evaluate life insurance applicants. Insurance industry standards were established because overweight people were poor insurance risks and were required to pay higher premiums, if they were offered coverage at all.

Although life insurance tables have become widely used, their utility in defining obesity has been questioned. One problem is that people with the lowest mortality rates tend to weigh less than the weight ranges given. Another problem is that insurance policy holders represent a select subset of the general population: they are largely white, middle-class adult males; and individuals with chronic disease or acute illnesses are often not included in life insurance statistics because they do not apply for insurance or are rejected. Also, body weights are often self-reported and inaccurate.

Despite these limitations, weight-for-height tables based on life insurance data are widely used because of their simplicity. The 1959 Metropolitan Life Desirable Weight Table (Society of Actuaries, 1959) has been used for years and continues to be the table of choice for many clinicians. As shown

TABLE 4.1 Desirable Weights for Men and Women Age 25 and Over

MEN							WOMEN			
HEIGHT		**FRAME**				**HEIGHT**		**FRAME**		
Feet	Inches	Small	Medium	Large		Feet	Inches	Small	Medium	Large
5	2	112–120	118–129	126–141		4	10	92–98	96–107	104–119
5	3	115–123	121–133	129–144		4	11	94–101	98–110	106–122
5	4	118–126	124–136	132–148		5	0	96–104	101–113	109–125
5	5	121–129	127–139	135–152		5	1	99–107	104–116	112–128
5	6	124–133	130–143	138–156		5	2	102–110	107–119	115–131
5	7	128–137	134–147	142–161		5	3	105–113	110–122	118–134
5	8	132–141	138–152	147–166		5	4	108–116	113–126	121–138
5	9	136–145	142–156	151–170		5	5	111–119	116–130	125–142
5	10	140–150	146–160	155–174		5	6	114–123	120–135	129–146
5	11	144–154	150–165	159–179		5	7	118–127	124–139	133–150
6	0	148–158	154–170	164–184		5	8	122–131	128–143	137–154
6	1	152–162	158–175	168–189		5	9	126–135	132–147	141–158
6	2	156–167	162–180	173–194		5	10	130–140	136–151	145–163
6	3	160–171	167–185	178–199		5	11	134–144	140–155	149–168
6	4	164–175	172–190	182–204		6	0	138–148	144–159	153–173

Source: Data adapted from the Statistical Bulletin, Metropolitan Life Insurance Company, New York. Derived primarily from data of the *1959 Build and Blood Pressure Study,* Society of Actuaries.

TABLE 4.4
Body Weight (in pounds) According to Height (in inches) and Body Mass Index

Body Mass Index (Body Weight)

Height	19	20	21	22	23	24	25	26	27	28	29	30	31	32	33	34	35	36	37	38	39	40	41	42	43	44	45	46	47	48	49	50
58	91	95	100	105	110	114	119	124	129	133	138	143	148	152	157	162	167	172	176	181	186	191	195	200	205	210	214	219	224	229	233	238
59	94	99	104	109	114	119	124	129	134	139	144	149	154	159	164	169	174	179	184	188	193	198	203	208	213	218	223	228	233	238	243	248
60	97	102	107	112	117	122	127	132	138	143	148	153	158	163	168	173	178	183	188	194	199	204	209	214	219	224	229	234	239	244	250	255
61	101	106	111	117	122	127	132	138	143	148	154	159	164	169	175	180	185	191	196	201	207	212	217	222	228	233	238	244	249	254	260	265
62	103	109	114	120	125	130	136	141	147	152	158	163	168	174	179	185	190	196	201	206	212	217	223	228	234	239	245	250	255	261	266	272
63	107	113	119	124	130	135	141	147	152	158	163	169	175	181	186	192	198	203	209	214	220	226	231	237	243	248	254	260	265	271	277	282
64	111	117	123	129	135	141	146	152	158	164	170	176	182	187	193	199	205	211	217	223	228	234	240	246	252	258	264	269	275	281	287	293
65	114	120	126	132	138	144	150	156	162	168	174	180	186	192	198	204	210	216	222	228	234	240	246	252	258	264	270	276	282	288	294	300
66	118	124	131	137	143	149	156	162	168	174	180	187	193	199	205	212	218	224	230	236	243	249	255	261	268	274	280	286	292	299	305	311
67	121	127	134	140	147	153	159	166	172	178	185	191	198	204	210	217	223	229	236	242	248	255	261	268	274	280	287	293	299	306	312	319
68	125	132	139	145	152	158	165	172	178	185	191	198	205	211	218	224	231	238	244	251	257	264	271	277	284	290	297	304	310	317	323	330
69	128	135	142	149	155	162	169	176	182	189	196	203	209	216	223	230	236	343	250	257	263	270	277	284	290	297	304	311	317	324	331	338
70	133	140	147	154	161	168	175	182	189	196	203	210	217	224	231	238	244	251	258	265	272	279	286	293	300	307	314	321	328	335	342	349
71	136	143	150	157	164	171	179	186	193	200	207	214	221	229	236	243	250	257	264	271	279	286	293	300	307	314	321	329	336	343	350	357
72	140	148	155	162	170	177	185	192	199	207	214	221	229	236	244	251	258	266	273	281	288	295	303	313	317	325	332	340	347	354	362	369
73	143	151	158	166	174	181	189	196	204	211	219	226	234	241	249	257	264	272	279	287	294	302	309	317	324	332	340	347	355	362	370	377
74	148	156	164	171	179	187	195	203	210	218	226	234	242	249	257	265	273	281	288	296	304	312	319	327	335	343	351	358	366	374	382	390
75	151	159	167	175	183	191	199	207	215	223	231	239	247	255	263	271	279	287	294	302	310	318	326	334	342	350	358	366	374	382	390	398
76	156	164	172	181	189	197	205	214	222	230	238	246	255	263	271	279	287	296	304	312	320	328	337	345	353	361	370	378	386	394	402	411

Source: Food and Nutrition Board, Institute of Medicine. (1995). *Weighing the Options: Criteria for Evaluating Weight-Management Programs.* Washington, D.C.: National Academy Press.

Thus:

$$\frac{165 \text{ pounds}}{143 \text{ pounds}} \times 100 = 115 \text{ percent}$$

This woman, then, has a relative weight of 115 percent. Generally, patients with a relative body weight of 120 percent to 129 percent are considered overweight; patients with a relative body weight of 130 percent to 199 percent or more are considered obese; and patients with a relative weight of 200 percent or more are considered severely obese.

Body Mass Index

Calculating BMI is another indirect method of estimating body fat content that is highly correlated with actual body fat content (Food and Nutrition Board, 1995). BMI (formerly known as Quetelet's index) is a mathematical ratio of weight to height:

$$BMI = \frac{\text{body weight (in kilograms)}}{\text{height}^2 \text{ (in meters)}}$$

To convert body weight in pounds to body weight in kilograms, multiply pounds by 0.45 (1 pound = 0.45 kilograms). To convert height in inches to height in meters, multiply inches by 0.0254 (1 inch = 0.0254 meters). *Table 4.4* simplifies these calculations by listing the BMI corresponding to various height and weight combinations.

To use the table, find the persons height in inches. The move horizontally across the table to find the person's body weight in pounds. The corresponding BMI across the top of each vertical row. For example, a man or woman measuring 68 inches tall and weighing 158 pounds would have a BMI of 24.

Based on 1959 Metropolitan Life Insurance Desirable Weight Table, a desirable BMI ranges from 20 to 25 for men and 19 to 26 for women. Based on the National Institutes of Health Task Force on Prevention and Treatment of Obesity (National Institute of Diabetes and Digestive and Kidney Diseases, 1993), individuals age 19 to 34 years old with a BMI greater than 25 are considered obese. Individuals ages 35 years and older with a BMI greater than 27 are considered obese. *Table 4.5* gives normal age-adjusted BMI levels, while *Table 4.6* lists BMI and degree of obesity.

Body Fat Distribution

In addition to body weight assessments using weight-for-height charts or BMI index, nurses should also assess the distribution of body fat. Excess fat deposits located in the upper body (abdominal or visceral area) are associated with greater health risks than fat deposited more in the lower body (gluteal area). Women tend to have more lower body obesity, yielding a pear shape,

TABLE 4.5
Body Mass Index, Normal Age-Adjusted Levels

Age range (yr.)	BMI (kg/m²)
19-24	19-24
25-34	20-25
35-44	21-26
45-54	21-26
55-64	23-28
65+	24-29

TABLE 4.6
Body Mass Index and Degree of Obesity

Degree of Obesity	BMI
Desirable weight	21-22
Overweight	25
Obesity	30
Medically significant obesity	35
Super obesity	40
Morbid obesity	45
Super morbid obesity	≥50

Source: National Institutes of Health Technology Assessment Conference. (1992). Methods for voluntary weight loss and control. *Annals of Internal Medicine* 116, 942–949.

while men tend to have more upper body obesity, yielding an apple shape.

The degree of upper or lower body obesity can be assessed using the waist-to-hip ratio as follows:

1. Use a nonstretchable tape measure to determine waist measurement at the smallest point between the rib cage and navel.

2. Determine hip measurement at the widest point around the buttocks.

3. Divide waist measurement by hip measurement to arrive at waist-to-hip ratio. A waist-to-hip ratio of greater than 1.0 for men and 0.8 for women indicates upper body obesity.

Figure 4.2 gives a nomogram for quick determination of waist-to-hip ratio.

DEFINING EATING DISORDERS

Fairburn and Walsh (1995) have defined an eating disorder as "a persistent disturbance of eating or eating-related behavior that results in the altered consumption or absorption of food and that significantly impairs physical health or psychosocial functioning." The eating disorder should not be secondary to other medical disorders or psychiatric disorders, such as Kleine-Levin syndromes, Prader-Willi syndrome, depression, mania, or dementia.

Although anorexia nervosa and bulimia nervosa are most commonly equated with the term

eating disorders, at least one-third of individuals with eating disorders fail to meet diagnostic criteria for either of these two disorders.

Thirty to forty years ago the eating disorder anorexia nervosa was thought to be a form of pituitary disease or a variant of other psychiatric disorders, such as depression, schizophrenia,

FIGURE 4.2 Nomogram for Determining Waist-to-Hip Ratio

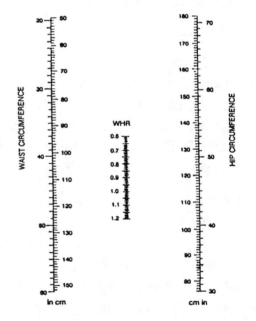

Place a ruler between the column for waist circumference and the column for hip circumference and read the ratio from the point where the ruler crosses the WHR line.

Source: Reprinted by permission of the *Western Journal of Medicine.* Bray, G. A., and D. S. Gray; Obesity: Part 1—Pathogenesis; 1988, volume 149, pages 429–441.

TABLE 4.7 DSM-IV Diagnostic Criteria for Anorexia Nervosa

A. Refusal to maintain body weight at or above a minimally normal weight for age and height (e.g., weight loss leading to maintenance of body weight less than 85% of that expected, or failure to make expected weight gain during period of growth, leading to body weight less than 85% of that expected).

B. Intense fear of gaining weight or becoming fat, even though underweight.

C. Disturbance in the way in which one's body weight or shape is experienced, undue influence of body weight or shape on self-evaluation, or denial of the seriousness of the current low body weight.

D. In postmenarchal females, amenorrhea, i.e., the absence of at least three consecutive menstrual cycles. (A woman is considered to have amenorrhea if her periods occur only following hormone, e.g., estrogen, administration).

Specify type:

Restricting Type: during the current episode of Anorexia Nervosa, the person has not regularly engaged in binge-eating or purging behavior (i.e., self-induced vomiting or the misuse of laxatives, diuretics, or enemas)

Binge-Eating/Purging Type: during the current episode of Anorexia Nervosa, the person has regularly engaged in binge-eating or purging behavior (i.e., self-induced vomiting or the misuse of laxatives, diuretics, or enemas)

Note: From American Psychiatric Association (1994). *Diagnostic and Statistical Manual of Mental Disorders* (4th ed., pp. 544-545). Washington, DC Author. Copyright 1994 by The American Psychiatric Association. Reprinted by permission.

obsessional disorder, or hysteria (Garfinkel, 1995). Since 1969, however, distinct criteria have been used to define anorexia nervosa. These criteria are based on both psychological and physiological signs and symptoms.

While bulimia has long been recognized as a symptom among people with anorexia nervosa, it has only been recognized as a distinct entity since the late 1970s. In more recent years binge-eating and atypical eating disorders have also been defined.

Anorexia Nervosa

Anorexia nervosa is characterized by behavior designed to produce significant weight loss, a morbid fear of becoming fat, and evidence of an endocrine disorder, such as missing menstrual periods for females or lack of sexual potency or interest in males. Both the American Psychiatric Association (1994) and the World Health Organization (1992) give specific diagnostic criteria for anorexia nervosa, as shown in *Tables 4.7 and 4.8.* The defining criteria of both of these associations are very similar.

Patients with anorexia nervosa are driven to be thin and refuse to maintain a minimally normal body weight (relative body weight of greater than 85 percent of desirable body weight). They have an intense fear of becoming fat and disturbed perception of their body image. They also have evidence of an endocrine disorder. Amenorrhea is a common feature of anorexia nervosa in females. The amenorrhea may be partly due to loss of body fat, but amenorrhea can also occur before the individual has lost much weight.

Some individuals with anorexia nervosa may binge on excessive amounts of foods and then purge themselves by self-induced vomiting or misuse of laxatives, diuretics, or enemas. Other individuals restrict their food intake without binging and purging, though they are often obsessed with food.

Bulimia Nervosa

While bulimia was once considered a variant of anorexia nervosa, bulimia nervosa is now considered a distinct clinical entity. As shown in *Tables 4.9 and 4.10,* bulimia nervosa is characterized by powerful and uncontrollable urges to overeat, purging to avoid the fattening effects of food, and a morbid fear of becoming fat.

Although there is some disagreement on what exactly constitutes a binge, patients with bulimia nervosa can consume unusually large amounts of foods in a short time period. Patients also have a feeling of loss of control while binging. For exam-

---

TABLE 4.8 ICD-10 Diagnostic Criteria for Anorexia Nervosa

For a definite diagnosis, all of the following are required:

(a) Body weight is maintained at least 15% below that expected (either lost or never achieved), or Quetelet's body-mass index is l7.5 or less. Prepubertal patients may show failure to make the expected weight gain during the period of growth.

(b) The weight loss is self-induced by avoidance of "fattening foods." One or more of the following may also be present: self-induced vomiting; self-induced purging; excessive exercise; use of appetite suppressants and/or diuretics.

(c) There is body-image distortion in the form of a specific psychopathology whereby a dread of fatness persists as an intrusive, overvalued idea and the patient imposes a low weight threshold on himself or herself.

(d) A widespread endocrine disorder involving the hypothalamic-pituitary-gonadal axis is manifest in women as amenorrhoea and in men as a loss of sexual interest and potency. (An apparent exception is the persistence of vaginal bleeds in anorexic women who are receiving replacement hormonal therapy, most commonly taken as a contraceptive pill.) There may also be elevated levels of growth hormone, raised levels of cortisol, changes in the peripheral metabolism of the thyroid hormone, and abnormalities of insulin secretion.

(e) If onset is prepubertal, the sequence of pubertal events is delayed or even arrested (growth ceases; in girls the breasts do not develop and there is a primary amenorrhoea; and in boys the genitals remain juvenile). With recovery, puberty is often completed normally, but the menarche is late.

Atypical Anorexia Nervosa: This term should be used for those individuals in whom one or more of the key features of anorexia nervosa, such as amenorrhoea or significant weight loss, is absent, but who otherwise present a fairly typical clinical picture. Such people are usually encountered in psychiatric liaison services in general hospitals or in primary care. Patients who have all the key symptoms but to only a mild degree may also be best described by this term. This term should not be used for eating disorders that resemble anorexia nervosa but that are due to known physical illness.

Note: From World Health Organization (1992). *The ICD-10 Classification of Mental and Behavioral Disorders: Clinical Descriptions and Diagnostic Guidelines* (pp. 176-181). Geneva: Author. Copyright 1992 by the World Health Organization. Reprinted by permission.

---

ple, it is not uncommon for patients with bulimia to eat a gallon or more of ice cream in 15 minutes, or two or three loaves of bread in less than a half an hour. In a survey of female outpatients with bulimia nervosa, deZwaan and Mitchell (1993) found that over 80 percent had a binge episode at least daily.

After, binging, patients try to compensate for the binge episode to avoid the fattening effects of food. Most patients (over 70 percent) purge through self-induced vomiting (deZwaan and Mitchell, 1993). Patients insert their fingers down their

---

TABLE 4.9 DSM-IV Diagnostic Criteria for Bulimia Nervosa

A. Recurrent episodes of binge-eating. An episode of binge-eating is characterized by both of the following:
    (1) eating, in a discrete period of time (e.g., within any 2-hour period), an amount of food that is definitely larger than most people would eat during a similar period of time and under similar circumstances
    (2) a sense of lack of control over eating during the episode (e.g., a feeling that one cannot stop eating or control what or how much one is eating)

B. Recurrent inappropriate compensatory behavior in order to prevent weight gain, such as self-induced vomiting; misuse of laxatives, diuretics, enemas, or other medications; fasting; or excessive exercise.

C. The binge-eating and inappropriate compensatory behaviors both occur, on average, at least twice a week for 3 months.

D. Self-evaluation is unduly influenced by body shape and weight.

E. The disturbance does not occur exclusively during episodes of Anorexia Nervosa.

Specify type:

Purging Type: during the current episode of Bulimia Nervosa, the person has regularly engaged in self-induced vomiting or the misuse of laxatives, diuretics, or enemas

Nonpurging Type: during the current episode of Bulimia Nervosa, the person has used other inappropriate compensatory behaviors, such as fasting or excessive exercise, but has not regularly engaged in self-induced vomiting or the misuse of laxatives, diuretics, or enemas

Note: From American Psychiatric Association (1994). *Diagnostic and Statistical Manual of Mental Disorders* (4th ed. pp. 549-550). Washington. DC: Author. Copyright 1994 by the American Psychiatric Association. Reprinted by permission.

TABLE 4.13 Research Criteria for Binge-Eating Disorder

A. Recurrent episodes of binge-eating. An episode of binge-eating is characterized by both of the following:
   (1) eating, in a discrete period of time (e.g., within any 2-hour period), an amount of food that is definitely larger than most people would eat in a similar period of time under similar circumstances; and
   (2) a sense of lack of control over eating during the episode (e.g., a feeling that one cannot stop eating or control what or how much one is eating).

B. The binge-eating episodes are associated with three (or more) of the following:
   (1) eating much more rapidly than normal
   (2) eating until feeling uncomfortably full
   (3) eating large amounts of food when not feeling physically hungry
   (4) eating alone because of being embarrassed by how much one is eating
   (5) feeling disgusted with oneself, depressed or very guilty after overeating

C. Marked distress regarding binge-eating is present.

D. The binge-eating occurs, on average, at least 2 days a week for 6 months.
   Note: The method of determining frequency differs from that used for Bulimia Nervosa; future research should address whether the preferred method of setting a frequency threshold is counting the number of days on which binges occur or counting the number of episodes of binge-eating.

E. The binge-eating is not associated with the regular use of inappropriate compensatory behaviors (e.g. purging, fasting, excessive exercise) and does not occur exclusively during the course of Anorexia Nervosa or Bulimia Nervosa.

Note: From American Psychiatric Association (1994). *Diagnostic and Statistical Manual of Mental Disorders* (4th ed. p. 731). Washington, DC: Author. Copyright 1994 by the American Psychiairic Association. Reprinted by permission.

EXAM QUESTIONS

CHAPTER 4
Questions 27–33

27. The term "overweight" means
    a. weighing up to 10 percent over recommended weight
    b. weighing up to 20 percent over recommended weight
    c. weighing up to 30 percent over recommended weight
    d. the same as the term "obese"

28. Body mass index is
    a. body weight in kilograms divided by height in meters squared
    b. body weight in kilograms squared divided by height in meters
    c. body weight in pounds divided by height in inches squared
    d. body weight in pounds squared divided by height in inches

29. The term "relative weight" refers to
    a. the ratio of an individual's body weight to the average weight of his or her parents
    b. actual body weight in pounds as a percentage of desirable body weight defined in weight-for-height tables
    c. body weight in kilograms divided by height in meters squared
    d. current body weight as a percentage of average body weight during the past year

30. Which of the following regarding weight-for-height tables is true?
    a. The 1959 and 1983 Metropolitan Life Insurance tables list comparable desirable body weights.
    b. The 1983 Metropolitan Life Insurance tables list lower desirable weights than the 1959 tables.
    c. The 1983 Metropolitan Life Insurance tables list higher desirable weights than the 1959 tables.
    d. The 1959 and 1983 Metropolitan Life Insurance tables are meant for different populations and are not comparable.

31. Which of the following is a diagnostic criteria for anorexia nervosa?
    a. amenorrhea or endocrine disorder
    b. hypotension
    c. depression
    d. obsessive-compulsive disorder

32. Which of the following is a diagnostic criteria for bulimia nervosa?
    a. regular self-induced vomiting
    b. amenorrhea or endocrine disorder
    c. body weight less than 85 percent of desirable weight
    d. recurrent episodes of binge-eating

33. Which of the following characteristics distinguishes diagnosis of individuals with bulimia nervosa from diagnosis of individuals with binge-eating disorder?

    a. depression

    b. binge episodes at least two days weekly for six months

    c. morbid fear of becoming fat

    d. pica of nonorganic origin

CHAPTER 5

ASSESSMENT OF PATIENTS WITH OBESITY OR EATING DISORDERS

CHAPTER OBJECTIVE

After studying this chapter, you will be able to describe the key elements of a comprehensive assessment of patients with obesity or eating disorders.

LEARNING OBJECTIVES

After studying this chapter, you will be able to

1. Recognize key elements of a baseline health history for patients with obesity or eating disorders.

2. Identify parts of the physical examination specific to assessment of obesity or eating disorders.

3. Specify alternative dietary assessment measures and indicate their uses.

4. Select laboratory tests indicated based on findings in the physical examination.

INTRODUCTION

Careful assessment of patients with obesity or eating disorder is essential to planning and implementing an effective course of treatment. A thorough medical and nutritional assessment should yield valuable information on the factors that cause or contribute to the weight problem, the existing level of medical and/or psychological risks, and the necessity of conducting further medical and laboratory evaluations. Just as treatment of obesity and eating disorders requires the expertise of a multidisciplinary health care team, so does assessment of these disorders.

The previous chapter defined obesity, anorexia nervosa, bulimia nervosa, and atypical eating disorders and gave criteria for diagnosis. This chapter describes elements of the health history, physical examination, diet history, and laboratory studies specific to assessment of obesity and eating disorders.

HEALTH HISTORY

In the initial interview, the nurse will want to obtain basic information about the patient, including a family health history and the patient's own health history. Most clinics use their own history-taking form, which acts as a baseline management summary.

The medical history should be focused on the specific eating disorder and should identify four factors (Weinsier, 1995):

- Factors contributing to obesity or the eating disorder

- Current medical complications

- Past treatments and responses

- Factors that would preclude weight intervention.

Assessment of factors that contribute to the weight or eating disorder should include familial, endocrine, behavioral, and psychosocial elements. In addition, nurses should also assess patients' attitudes toward their body weight and shape.

For assessment of obesity, the initial health history should include questions on

- Family history of obesity and related health problems

- The patient's health history, especially incidence of high blood lipids, high blood pressure, glucose intolerance, diabetes, cancer, osteoarthritis, and other problems potentially related to obesity

- Age of onset of obesity

- Weight history, including significant weight fluctuations

- Past obesity treatment attempts and responses

Pregnancy, lactation, or a history of anorexia nervosa are factors that would preclude initiating a weight-loss program. For children and older adults, benefits of attempting weight control must be carefully weighed against risks (see Chapter 11, Intervention: Management of Obesity and Eating Disorders in Special Populations).

Table 5.1 summarizes factors to be considered when taking a health history of an obese patient. A general sample health history form is shown in *Figure 5.1,* which can be modified as needed.

For assessment of eating disorders, nurses should focus more attention on weight history,

---

TABLE 5.1 Factors to Be Considered When Taking a Health History of an Obese Patient

Factors predisposing to/associated with obesity
Family history of obesity (number of first-degree relatives who are obese)
Age of onset
In children: growth pattern, mental and physical maturation
Potential endocrine abnormalities
> *Hypothyroidism:* symptoms include cold intolerance, menstrual abnormalities, constipation, weakness
> *Cushing's syndrome:* symptoms include hypertension, glucose intolerance, menstrual dysfunction, weakness, back pain, compression fractures, bruising
> *Polycystic ovarian syndrome:* symptoms include reduced/absent menses shortly after menarche, hirsutism
Life-style changes concurrent with onset of weight gain (e.g., job change, marriage/divorce, childbirth, relocation)
Dietary pattern (best reviewed with diet records)
Pattern of physical activity (best reviewed with exercise records)

History of medical complications of obesity
Cancer (especially of endometrium and breast)
Glucose intolerance and diabetes mellitus
Hepatobiliary disease (especially gallstones, hepatic steatosis and enlargement)
Hypertension, hyperlipidemia, coronary artery disease
Osteoarthritis (especially, but not exclusively, of weight-bearing joints)
Respiratory disease (especially periodic apnea due to obstruction, or alveolar hypoventilation)

Previous treatment responses
Past successes, failures; weight-cycling pattern
Past medical and surgical therapies for obesity

Factors warranting precaution/precluding weight reduction
<20 or >65 years of age
History of anorexia nervosa
Pregnancy or lactation

Source: Weinsier, R. L. (1995). Clinical assessment of obese patients. In K. D. Brownell, & C. G. Fairburn, (Eds.). *Eating disorders and obesity,* (pp. 463–468). New York: The Guilford Press.

FIGURE 5.1 Sample Health History for an Obese Patient

BASELINE MANAGEMENT SUMMARY

Patient's name _____

Date _____

Marital status
☐ Single ☐ Married ☐ Divorced ☐ Widowed

Patient's Characteristics and Health Habits
Age_____ Sex_____ Height_____

Weight_____% of ideal weight_____
Impairments that would affect dietary change or
counseling _____

FAMILY MEDICAL HISTORY

Is the patient's father living? ☐ Yes ☐ No ☐ Unsure
If not, at what age did he die?

Cause _____

Is the patient's mother living? ☐ Yes ☐ No ☐ Unsure
If not, at what age did she die?

Cause _____

How many brothers and sisters does patient have?_____

How many are living?_____

Do or did any of the brothers or sisters, mother or father,
have any of the following medical problems? (Use M for
mother, F for father, S for sister, B for brother.)

Hypertension _____

Diabetes _____

Overweight_____

Stroke _____

Hyperlipidemia _____

Type _____

Diet prescription_____

Does the spouse have a weight problem? ☐ Yes ☐ No

Describe the problem:_____

_____

Hypertension ☐ Yes ☐ No
Diabetes ☐ Yes ☐ No
Premature heart attack ☐ Yes ☐ No
Stroke ☐ Yes ☐ No
Hyperlipidemia ☐ Yes ☐ No

Type _____

Diet prescription _____

PATIENT'S MEDICAL HISTORY

Lowest adult weight _____

Highest adult weight _____

Does the patient have any evidence of cardiovascular disease? ☐ Yes ☐ No

Date_____

Describe _____

_____

Hyperlipoproteinemia? ☐ Yes ☐ No

Type _____

Lipid-lowering medications _____

Hypertension? ☐ Yes ☐ No

Medications_____

Potassium supplement _____

Uric acid medications_____

Diabetes? ☐ Yes ☐ No

Medications_____

Hypothyroidism? ☐ Yes ☐ No

Medications_____

Kidney disease? ☐ Yes ☐ No
Liver disease? ☐ Yes ☐ No

Medications_____

Alcohol abuse? ☐ Yes ☐ No
Taking corticosteroids? ☐ Yes ☐ No
Taking oral contraceptives? ☐ Yes ☐ No
ECG changes or positive stress test? ☐ Yes ☐ No
Taking nonprescription drugs? ☐ Yes ☐ No

Kind _____

Adapted from: National Institutes of Health (1987). *Heart to Heart, A Manual on Nutrition. Counseling for the Reduction of Cardiovascular Disease Risk Factors*. Bethesda, MD. p.26.

Baseline Blood Values   Date

Total cholesterol   _____   _____

LDL cholesterol   _____   _____

VLDL cholesterol   _____   _____

HDL cholesterol   _____   _____

Triglycerides   _____   _____

Glucose   _____   _____

Uric acid   _____   _____

Potassium   _____   _____

Other: _____

Baseline blood pressure:____/____ _____

Other Characteristics

Does patient live with: ☐ Family ☐ Friends ☐ Alone

Patient's occupation: _____

Hours per week_____ Shift work?_____

Occupations of others in household: _____

_____

_____

_____

_____

Household income level: ☐ Low ☐ Middle ☐ High

Receiving assistance? _____

Patient's education:
Finished high school? ☐ Yes ☐ No
Finished college? ☐ Yes ☐ No
Does patient speak English? ☐ Yes ☐ No

Other _____

Does patient read English? ☐ Yes ☐ No

Other _____

Does patient have a seeing, hearing, or other impairment? ☐ Yes ☐ No
Specify _____

If yes, does patient have a friend or relative who can assist? _____

Health Habits and Lifestyle

1. Smoking:
    ☐ Smokes cigarettes
    ☐ Number smoked per day_____
    ☐ Smokes pipe/cigars
    ☐ Nonsmoker
    ☐ Quit smoking during the past year

2. Physical activity (include any activity on the job)

	Minutes/day	**Times/week**
Walking	_____	_____
Jogging	_____	_____
Swimming	_____	_____
Bicycling	_____	_____
Other:	_____	_____

Specify _____

3. Does patient seem to be a time-oriented, stressed, or very structured person? ☐ Yes ☐ No

4. Has the patient had any severe personal problems in the past 12 months? (For example, death of a family member, marital problems, divorce, lawsuits, job change, serious problems with children, accidents, or evidence of alcohol or drug abuse?)

5. Will family members support the need for changing food habits? ☐ Yes ☐ No

Comments: _____

_____

_____

_____

_____

_____

_____

body image, and means of weight control—including purging behaviors such as vomiting and use of laxatives, drugs, or excessive exercise—during the health history (Kaplan and Garfinkle, 1993).

Assessment of weight history should include current weight, highest weight ever, lowest weight ever, usual weight before the eating disorder developed, weight at which abnormal menstrual function (if any) occurred, and the patients' own image of what his or her ideal weight should be. The greater the gap between perceived ideal weight and ideal weight according to established weight-for-height charts, the greater the severity of the eating disorder. Likewise, the greater the patient's dissatisfaction with body weight and the more negative the patient's body image, the greater the severity of the eating disorder.

Patients with eating disorders are often embarrassed about their eating and purging behaviors and very reluctant to discuss these behaviors. The nurse will have to ask specific questions for comprehensive assessment of such behaviors.

Eating behaviors can be assessed with a diet history, as described in a following section of this chapter. Nurses should ask specific questions about the frequency, timing, and preceding events associated with episodes of binge-eating. Food phobias and preoccupations also need to be discussed.

Nurses should also ask whether patients ever induce vomiting to purge themselves. The majority of patients with bulimia vomit to purge themselves, many at least once daily. About 25 percent of patients with anorexia nervosa vomit regularly (Kaplan and Garfinkel, 1993). If the patient induces vomiting, frequency and method should be determined. Nurses should specifically ask whether the patient uses or has ever used syrup of ipecac to induce vomiting.

Individuals with eating disorders also use laxatives or drugs to purge themselves. Nurses should ask whether the patient uses any of the following:

- Laxatives
- Diet pills
- Diuretics
- Caffeine
- Thyroid medications

Questions on frequency and intensity of exercise should also be included.

Table 5.2 gives specific factors to be included in assessment of individuals with eating disorders. *Table 5.3* gives sample interview questions for the diagnosis of eating disorders. Another instrument, the Eating Disorders Examination (Fairburn and Cooper, 1993), is a semi-structured interview that is considered the "gold standard" for assessing specific symptoms of eating disorders (Garner, 1995). This instrument can be used to diagnose eating disorders and permits the interviewer to clarify the meaning of patients' responses. Disadvantages of the Eating Disorders Examination, however, are that it takes about one hour to administer, requires a trained interviewer, and is not suitable for group administration.

Since many patients with both obesity and eating disorders have associated depression, anxiety, disturbances in relationships, or substance abuse, nurses and other health professionals can also assess the incidence and severity of these problems. *Table 5.4* lists specific questions relating to these problems that can be included in assessment of patients with eating disorders.

PHYSICAL EXAMINATION

Once the nurse has obtained a comprehensive health history, a thorough physical examination should be performed. Physical examination usually begins with measurement of weight and height. Patients with obesity and eating disorders often self-report body weight inaccurately, so an accurate measurement must be taken. Current body weight can be compared to recommended weights established in weight-for-height tables, as described in chapter four. For obese individuals, the distribution of body fat should also be assessed by comparing waist-to-hip ratio, as described in chapter four.

Body mass index (BMI) is highly correlated with actual body fat content and provides a very helpful means of expressing body fatness or thin-

TABLE 5.2 Factors to be Considered When Assessing a Patient with an Eating Disorder

I. Weight
   A. Current (BMI)
   B. Highest ever
   C. Lowest ever
   D. Premorbid
   E. Perceived ideal
   F. Menstrual threshold

II. Body Image
   A. Attitudes and feelings re: overall size
   B. Attitudes and feelings re: specific body parts
   C. Cosmetic procedures

III. Means of Weight Control
   A. Caloric Intake
      1. Number of calories
      2. Number of meals
      3. Binge episodes
         a. Frequency
         b. Time of day or night
         c. Amount of food consumed
         d. Type of food consumed
         e. Subjective experience
         f. Associated behaviors—stealing, rumination, pica
      4. Idiosyncratic nutritional beliefs and practices
   B. Purging behaviors
      1. Vomiting (ipecac)
      2. Laxatives
      3. Drugs to control weight
         a. Diet pills
         b. Diuretics
         c. Caffeine
         d. Thyroid
   C. Exercise
      1. Type
      2. Amount

IV. Physical and Laboratory Examination
   A. Review of systems (especially cardiovascular, gastrointestinal, endocrine, gynecologic, dermatologic)
   B. Physical complications
   C. Laboratory investigations
      1. Routine
         a. CBC
         b. Electrolytes
         c. BUN
         d. Creatinine
      2. If indicated
         a. EKG (weight loss, hypokalemia, ipecac)
         b. Liver function (weight loss, alcohol abuse)
         c. CPK (abusing ipecac)
         d. Amylase (gastrointestinal symptoms)
         e. Calcium, phosphorus (chronic amenorrhea or fractures)
         f. Endoscopic or roentgenographic exam (blood loss)

V. Initial feedback
   A. Cessation of dieting behavior
   B. Regular intake of adequate calories (2,000–3,000 calories/day)
   C. Proscription of laxatives, diet pills, diuretics
   D. If underweight, cessation of exercise

VI. Medical indications for immediate hospitalization
   A. Severe fluid and electrolyte disturbance (i.e., K <2.5 m mol/L)
   B. Cardiac complications
      1. Arrhythmia or conduction disturbance (i.e., QT prolongation)
      2. Cardiomyopathy (ipecac)
   C. Acute rapid weight loss
   D. Acute pancreatitis or gastric dilatation
   E. Convulsions

VII. Ongoing medical management
   A. Close monitoring of weight, fluid and electrolyte and cardiac status
   B. Psychiatric consultation
   C. Dental consultation
   D. Nutrition consultation
   E. Periodic hospitalization
      1. Crisis intervention for medical or psychiatric reasons
      2. In a specialized unit to treat the eating disorder

Source: Kaplan, A. S., & Garfinkle, P. E. (1993). *Medical issues and the eating disorders: the interface.* New York: Brunner/Mazel Publishers.

TABLE 5.3 Sample Interview Questions for the Diagnosis of Eating Disorders

DATE _____ NAME _____ AGE _____ RACE _____

DATE OF BIRTH_____ WEIGHT_____ HEIGHT _____

ADDRESS _____

TELEPHONE_____ REFERRED BY _____

I.   *General Assessment and History*

    1.   What types of problems do you have with eating or weight-related matters? How long has this been a problem?

    2.   What has been your highest and lowest weight? When?

    3.   Were you overweight as a child?   Y   N   (Describe.)

    4.   Were you/are you overweight as an adolescent?   Y   N   (Describe.)

    5.   What has been the course of your eating problems? (How the behavior began, increases, decreases, changes in eating.)

    6.   Have you had any medical/dental problems? (Check for dizziness, LBP, HBP, tooth erosion, thyroid problems, diabetes.)

    7.   Do you avoid eating certain foods?   Y   N   (Describe.)

        What emotional reaction occurs when you eat these "forbidden" foods? (Foods which are avoided or purged due to a belief that the foods will lead to rapid and significant weight gain.)

    8.   How many members are there in your household?

        Do they know about your eating problems?   Y   N

        If yes, how do they react/feel about your eating disorder?

        Would they participate in your treatment?

II. *Anorexia Nervosa*

    1.   Do you currently go periods of time without eating (starvation) to control your weight?   Y   N   (If Y, describe.)

        When did you first begin to lose weight/restrict your eating?

        Are there any factors/situations which seem to increase or decrease periods of restrictive eating?

TABLE 5.3 Sample Interview Questions for the Diagnosis of Eating Disorders *(Cont.)*

2. Do you feel that your weight is normal?   Y   N   (Describe.)

3. What emotional reaction would you have if you lost

   2 lbs.?

   5 lbs.?

   10 lbs.?

   What emotional reaction would you have if you gained

   2 lbs.?

   5 lbs.?

   10 lbs.?

4. Do you wish to be thinner than you are now?   Y   N   (If Y, ask what body areas should be thinner.)

   What is your goal weight?

   Do you think or worry a lot about your weight and body size?

   Do you often feel "fat" when you gain only a few pounds?   Y   N   (Describe.)

   Do you weigh yourself often?   Y   N   How often?

5. When was your last menstrual cycle?

   Have you experienced menstrual irregularities within the last three months?   Y   N   (Describe.)

III. *Bulimia Nervosa*

1. Do you ever binge (rapid consumption of large amounts of food in a discrete period of time)? What is the daily course of your binge-eating? (Describe all covert and overt events that usually occur prior to, during, and after a binge.)

   Do you ever feel as though you have overeaten when you eat small portions of certain fattening foods?   Y   N   (Describe.)

   When did you first begin to have problems with binging?

   Are there any factors which appear to increase or decrease the frequency of binge-eating?

2. Do you feel out of control prior to or during a binge?   Y   N   (Describe.)

   Do you feel hungry prior to a binge?   Y   N

3. Do you purge after meals or after a binge?   Y   N

   Do you vomit?   Y   N   How often per day/week?

TABLE 5.3 Sample Interview Questions for the Diagnosis of Eating Disorders *(Cont.)*

Do you use laxatives?   Y   N   How often, what type?

Do you use diuretics?   Y   N   How often, what type?

Do you use appetite suppressants?   Y   N   How often, what type?

Do you often go on strict diets?   Y   N   How often, what type?

Do you engage in vigorous exercise?   Y   N   How often, what type?

When did you first begin to purge?

Are there any factors which appear to increase or decrease the frequency of purging?

4. How often does the binge-eating occur?

How long have you been binging at least twice per week?

How often does the binge-purge cycle occur?

IV. *Compulsive Overeating*

1. If you binge, what types of food do you typically eat?

2. Do you binge alone, or in secret?   Y   N   (Describe.)

3. What emotions typically precede a binge?

4. Do you often attempt to diet in order to lose weight? (Describe.)

5. Have you had frequent weight fluctuations greater than 10 pounds in the past few years?   Y   N   (Describe.)

6. Do you consider your eating to be abnormal?   Y   N

Do you feel that you have control over your eating?   Y   N

7. How do you feel during and after a binge episode? (Describe.)

8. Are you satisfied with your current weight?   Y   N   If no, what is your weight goal?

Source: Williamson, D.A. (1990). *Assessment of eating disorders.* New York: Pergamon Press.

ness. As shown in *Table 5.5,* health risks of obesity increase with increasing BMI. Risks are greater when other obesity-related health problems are pre-

sent or when waist-to-hip ratio is elevated.

Other parts of the physical exam include blood pressure (taken with the correct sized cuff); exami-

TABLE 5.4 Sample Interview Questions Relating to Depression, Anxiety, Relationships, and Substance Abuse

MOOD How have you been feeling lately? What has your mood been like? Have you been worried or upset? Have you felt any anxiety or panic (describe symptoms)?

If patient reports anxiety symptoms, ask the following question: Does the anxiety occur at any particular time, place or situation? Are there any situations you avoid because they make you nervous or scared?

SLEEP Do you have trouble falling asleep? Do you wake often during the night? Do you wake early in the morning before you would like to? Can you get back to sleep? Are you sleeping more than usual? How much? Do you usually take naps during the day? For how long?

SOMATIC/APPETITE Have you noticed any changes in your body lately? Have you been constipated? Have you noticed changes in your heart rate or breathing? How has your appetite been? Have you had trouble eating? Is this related to your mood?

OBSESSIVE-COMPULSIVE Have you had trouble with your thoughts? Do you ever have thoughts that bother you but you can't seem to get rid of them? Do you ever seem compelled to do something? Do you have any ritualistic habits (give examples)?

ACTIVITY/INTEREST Has it been hard to go out and do things lately? Do you have to push yourself? Do you seem to tire easily? Are you as interested in things as you used to be? Do you get as much pleasure out of things as you used to? Is there anything that you still enjoy?

HOPELESSNESS Do you think that things will get better? What does the future look like? Does anything lift your spirits or encourage you anymore?

WORTHLESSNESS How do you feel about yourself? Do you have a tendency to get down on yourself? What is your self-esteem like? Do you like yourself? Do you ever feel like a failure? How much of the time?

CONCENTRATION Have you had trouble concentrating lately? Have you been forgetting things? Have you had trouble making decisions recently?

SUICIDE Do you feel like life is worth living right now? Have you thought much about death? Have you considered taking your life?

RELATIONSHIPS
Do you like to do things with friends? How often? How many close friends would you say that you have? Are you experiencing any problems with your friends?

Are you married? Are you dating someone regularly? Is this area of your life going well? Would you like it to improve? Are you experiencing any other problems with relatives?

SUBSTANCE USE
Do you like to drink alcohol? How much do you usually drink? How often?

Do you take any prescription or nonprescription drugs? What type? How often?

Has your use of alcohol or drugs ever gotten you into any trouble? Have you ever experienced a blackout? Have you ever received a DWI or DUI? Have you ever received treatment for drug or alcohol related problems?

Source: Williamson, D.A. (1990). *Assessment of eating disorders.* New York: Pergamon Press.

nation of the skin; determination of body fat distribution; examination of the thyroid gland; examination for the presence of edema; neurologic examination; and a review of all body systems—especially cardiovascular, gastrointestinal, endocrine, gynecologic, and dermatologic. The physical examination should rule out endocrine disorders such as hypothyroidism, Cushing's syndrome, or polycystic ovarian syndrome.

Patients with eating disorders are often reluctant to admit the problem and first present to a medical establishment with some other complaint. Common physical signs found in patients with eating disorders include bilateral parotid gland enlargement, calluses on the dorsum of the hand from repeated self-induced vomiting, petechiae, irritation around the mouth from stomach acid, thinning of the scalp hair, lanugo hair growth, and a yellowish hue to the skin (Kaplan and Garfinkle, 1993). Chapter three also reviews the medical complications common in patients with eating disorders. *Figure 5.6* lists physical signs of good and poor nutrition to be assessed during the physical examination.

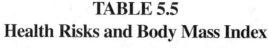

TABLE 5.5
Health Risks and Body Mass Index

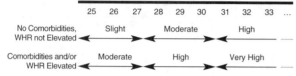

Body Mass Index (BMI)

	25	26	27	28	29	30	31	32	33	...
No Comorbidities, WHR not Elevated	Slight			Moderate			High			
Comorbidities and/or WHR Elevated	Moderate			High			Very High			

The risks are increased when adipose tissue is concentrated in the abdominal or visceral region (which is clinically assessed by calculating the waist-to-hip ratio [>1.0 for males and >0.8 for females]) and the presence of comorbidities such as high blood pressure (>140/90), lipid concentrations (cholesterol >200 mg/dl; triglycerides >225 mg/dl), non-insulin-dependent diabetes mellitus, osteoarthritis, sleep apnea, and premature death in the family from coronary heart disease. This figure presents general guidelines; each obese person requires individual evaluation.

Source: Food and Nutrition Board, Institute of Medicine. (1995). *Weighing the Options: Criteria for Evaluating Weight-management Programs.* Washington, D.C.: National Academy Press.

DIETARY ASSESSMENT

Dietary assessment should reveal usual eating patterns, types and quantities of foods eaten, and information about the eating environment such as food-related thoughts and eating cues. A registered dietitian will often be responsible for dietary assessment of the obese patient. A careful history of diet and nutritional information in relation to the patient's living situation and other personal, psychosocial, and economic problems, is another essential part of the nutritional assessment of any patient. isn't always easy to get accurate information. Many overweight persons aren't really aware of everything they are eating. Most people have no idea how many calories they consume during an average day, and many fool themselves into thinking they are being careful and cutting back, not taking into account the late-night refrigerator raids.

Food Records

A food record (also called a diet diary) kept for 24 hours or longer can give patients and their health care professionals a better idea of actual food consumption. A diet diary, kept for 24 hours or longer, can give a clearer picture of what they're really eating. Having a patient monitor his or her eating habits will accomplish three things: It will help the patient (1) become aware of his own behavior, such as eating too much late at night; (2) set goals for change, for example, substituting lower-calorie snacks for heavy dinners; and (3) find ways to reinforce or support the new behavior (Simonson, 1983).

Awareness of food problems begins with the patient's participation in the first assessment. It continues with the patient learning to observe his own behavior throughout the counseling period and keeping records.

Record-keeping or self-monitoring by the patient can be an important way to help him achieve long-term behavioral changes. A detailed food diary is very useful at the beginning, and at differing times throughout the diet. In some cases, it is helpful to have a prospective patient keep a three-day food diary before he or she comes in the first time.

Why keep a food diary? Self-monitoring can help the patient in many ways:

1. It can provide information about eating habits and the factors that influence them.

2. It helps the patient get involved in observing and analyzing his own diet habits.

3. It increases the patient's awareness of his diet and behavior.

4. It gives the health practitioner and patient something to review objectively and impartially—they can focus on problems on the record, not on the patient.

5. It reinforces new behavior, and serves as a reminder that allows the individual to make corrections. For example, a patient may find he is consuming too many high-calorie beverages, so he may decide to switch to sugar-free iced tea, colas, coffee, or water.

6. It increases the patient's skill in manipulating

TABLE 5.6 Physical Signs of Good Nutrition

General appearance:
Good nutrition: Alert, responsive, energetic, good endurance, sleeps well, vigorous
Poor nutrition: Listless, apathetic, cachexia, easily fatigued, no energy, falls asleep easily, looks tired, apathetic

Weight:
Good nutrition: Weight normal for height, age, and body build
Poor nutrition: Overweight or underweight

Posture:
Good nutrition: Erect posture, arms and legs straight
Poor nutrition: Sagging shoulders, sunken chest, humped back

Muscles:
Good nutrition: Well developed, firm, good tone, some fat under skin
Poor nutrition: Flaccid, poor tone, underdeveloped, tender, "wasted" appearance, cannot walk properly

Nervous system:
Good nutrition: Good attention span, not irritable or restless, normal reflexes, psychological stability
Poor nutrition: Inattentive, irritable, confused, paresthesias, loss of position and vibratory sense, weakness and tenderness of muscles, decreased or lost ankle and knee reflexes

Gastrointestinal function:
Good nutrition: Good appetite and digestion, normal regular elimination, no palpable organs or masses
Poor nutrition: Anorexia, indigestion, constipation or diarrhea, liver or spleen enlargement

Cardiovascular function:
Good nutrition: Normal heart rate and rhythm, no murmurs, blood pressure normal for age
Poor nutrition: Rapid heart rate (above 100 beats per minute), enlarged heart, abnormal rhythm, elevated blood pressure

Hair:
Good nutrition: Shiny, lustrous, firm, not easily pulled out, healthy scalp
Poor nutrition: Stringy, dull, brittle, dry, thin and sparse, depigmented, can be easily pulled out

Overall skin condition:
Good nutrition: Smooth, slightly moist, good color
Poor nutrition: Rough, dry, scaly, pale, pigmented, irritated, bruises, petechiae

Face and neck:
Good nutrition: Skin color uniform, smooth, pink, with a healthy appearance and not swollen
Poor nutrition: Greasy, discolored, scaly, swollen, dark skin over cheeks and under eyes, lumpiness or flakiness of skin around nose and mouth

Lips:
Good nutrition: smooth, good color, moist, not chapped or swollen
Poor nutrition: Dry, scaly, swollen, redness and swelling (cheilosis) or angular lesions at corners of the mouth or fissures or scars (stomatitis)

Mouth, oral membranes:
Good nutrition: Reddish pink mucous membranes in oral cavity
Poor nutrition: Swollen, boggy oral mucous membranes

Gums:
Good nutrition: Good pink color, healthy, red, no swelling or bleeding
Poor nutrition: Spongy, bleed easily, marginal redness, inflamed, gums receding

Tongue:
Good nutrition: Good pink color or deep reddish in appearance, not swollen or smooth, surface papillae present, no lesion
Poor nutrition: Swelling, scarlet and raw, magenta color, glossitis, hyperemic and hypertrophic papillae, atrophic papillae

Teeth:
Good nutrition: No cavities, no pain, bright, straight, no crowding, well-shaped jaw, clean, no discoloration
Poor nutrition: Unfilled cavities, absent teeth, worn surfaces, mottled (fluorosis), malpositioned

Eyes:
Good nutrition: Bright, clear, shiny, no sores at corners of eyelids, membranes moist and a healthy pink color, no prominent blood vessels or mount of tissue or sclera, no fatigue circles underneath eyes
Poor nutrition: Pale conjunctivas, conjunctival injection, dryness, signs of infection, Bitot's spots, redness and fissuring of eyelid corners, dryness of eye membrane, dull appearance of cornea (corneal xerosis), soft cornea (keratomalacia)

Neck:
Good nutrition: No enlargement of glands
Poor nutrition: Thyroid enlarged

Nails:
Good nutrition: Firm, pink
Poor nutrition: Brittle, ridged, spoon-shaped

Legs, feet:
Good nutrition: No tenderness, weakness, or swelling, good color
Poor nutrition: Edema, tender calf, tingling weakness

Skeleton:
Good nutrition: No malformations
Poor nutrition: Bowlegs, knock-knees, chest deformity at diaphragm, beaded ribs, prominent scapulas

the diet to achieve desired results. For example, the patient may find a variety of low-fat animal and vegetable protein sources, or find acceptable snack foods that fit into the daily food pattern.

7. It increases interaction between the health prac-

titioner and patient.

When counseling a patient, it is essential to know the patient's usual diet pattern. Having the patient keep a three-day food diary (some use a week-long, or even a 14-day form), provides a baseline for planning and measuring later changes.

Be sure to have a well-designed form ready at the first meeting, and ask the patient to start keeping records soon afterwards. Depending on what is being assessed, the diary may include types and amounts of food eaten, the location, time of day, time spent eating, what else the patient was doing at the same time, such as watching television or reading. Was the patient with anyone, and what was the overall mood at the time of eating? For patients with eating disorders, mood, bingeing and purging activity can also be recorded.

The diary can have many forms, including exercise data. It should include most of the following information:

1. Type of day—workday or nonworkday

2. Place food was eaten and the circumstances—at home or away, during a party, in a restaurant, etc.

3. The kind of food eaten

4. The time food was eaten

5. The amount eaten, as accurately as possible

6. How the food was prepared

Some also include suggestions to patients for completing food records. The following are suggested by the NIH (1987):

1. Records should include all meals any time of the day or night, snacks, coffee breaks, soft drink breaks, cocktails, beer, anything you nibble, every refrigerator raid.

2. Try to write down any foods immediately in the food record.

The following questions are particularly important in regard to high-fat foods or cholesterol-con-

taining foods:

3. Were fats or oils used in cooking or baking? If so, what brands were used?

4. Did you use salad dressings or mayonnaise in salads or on sandwiches?

5. Did you add fat to vegetables while cooking or afterward? If so, what kind did you add?

6. What kind of milk did you drink or use in cooking?

7. Did you eat margarine or butter on bread, toast, sandwiches, rolls, potatoes, etc.? If you used margarine, what brand did you choose?

8. Were gravies, sauces, or syrups added to any of your foods?

9. What cuts of meat were eaten? Did you trim off the fat or not?

10. What ingredients were used in mixed dishes, sandwiches, etc.?

11. Record in ounces all beverages, including alcoholic beverages.

12. Be sure to include how many and what size bread, rolls, crackers, raw fruits and vegetables, cookies, candies, snack items, etc.

13. Record by servings and size: pie, cake, coffee cake

14. Record in cups or by servings: potatoes, rice, fruits, vegetables, cereals, soups, casseroles.

15. Record in teaspoons or tablespoons any jellies, jams, sugar, syrup, sauces, gravies, salad dressings, butter, margarine, nuts, and seeds.

Some programs also include a snack record form that the patient can carry in pocket or purse, to record foods eaten away from home. This record should also include the day, the time of day, whether the food was eaten while the person was alone or with someone (list the person), the type of food eaten, and the amount eaten.

Accuracy is important. It is vital to emphasize to the patient that accuracy is important. Select methods that are easy to use, convenient, and readily available when the behavior occurs. Some encourage the patient to make suggestions on what to record as well as how to do so. For example, the patient may find it easier to carry a pocket-sized food diary with her at all times, or attach a "breakfast record" to the refrigerator, or keep a list of evening snacks on the dresser.

Keep instructions clear. Make sure the patient understands the purpose of keeping the food diary. Also, go over any form or any part of the form that might be confusing, or, if in doubt, have the patient fill out a sample page. If asked to record amounts of food, make sure the patient knows how to estimate amounts of food, and has a good food scale and measuring cups and spoons at home. Use familiar household measurements with cups and spoons or food models, to relate portions to familiar shapes and sizes. It's good to be specific about sizes and portions; an apple, for example, may be small or so large it takes two hands to hold it— quite a difference in calories!

Be sure the records the patient is keeping are relevant to the dietary problem at hand. Don't ask for more information than needed, and stress that the patient need only keep records if the information is useful.

Encourage the patient to make prompt notations about eating. Nothing is more frustrating than trying to remember what one had for lunch when it's dinnertime.

Use the records to observe patterns, not to judge behavior. Avoid expressing disapproval. Remember, many people are reluctant to reveal their full eating habits, especially if they seem embarrassing or unhealthy. Not many persons want to admit eating a half-gallon of rocky road ice cream or two tubs of popcorn, or fasting one day to gorge the next. Instead, whatever the eating habits may be, the purpose of the diary is to help both nurse and patient accurately assess the patient's current diet, plan changes, and identify problem eating behaviors. Records are only an aid, not a judgment. The records should be as complete as possible, and should include even tiny portions of food, such as half a tablespoonful, or just a bite. It all adds up.

The diet diary may reveal some surprising things. A person who feels she is eating like a bird may actually be tasting and sampling food, all day long, and eating far more calories than she would if she ate three moderate meals. Or a man who eats a light breakfast and lunch may be defeating himself by eating a calorie-laden dinner and snacking steadily into the late-evening hours.

For food records to be useful and accurate, patients must pay careful attention to estimating portion size. To increase accuracy, the health professional can ask patients to weigh and measure foods for a few days or anytime they are unsure of portion sizes. A recent study by Lichtman and colleagues (1992) found that some obese subjects who reported difficulty losing weight on a low-calorie diet underreported calorie intake by almost 50 percent.

It is important to use the information gained from a patient's food diaries, especially if he or she has faithfully kept a diary. By reviewing the records together, health professionals can teach patients about foods that are high in cholesterol or fat. These records can also show the patient's problem areas; for example, extra-large portions of high-fat foods, or lack of vegetables.

A food diary can be invaluable for patients because it allows them to use self-monitoring, an important means of continuing to assess the diet and measure change. Encouraging the patient to be involved in assessment and self-observation is a good strategy of beginning, promoting, and helping him adhere to the diet.

Self-monitoring tends to change behavior through the development of an increased awareness of self, and tends to do this in a favorable direction. Self-monitoring also has an important second benefit: It serves as a reminder which allows the patient to take self-corrective action.

Twenty-Four-Hour Food Recall

For some patients, keeping records simply is not feasible. Some persons aren't willing to take the time needed to fill out a regular diet diary. Others are unable to do so because of language difficulties or problems with reading and writing. There are other ways to get the information, such as having the patient call in on a regular basis to give a 24-hour recall of foods eaten, or asking the patient to complete a food checklist (see below), or simply continuing to ask pertinent questions about how well he is doing if he is trying to change certain diet patterns.

To take a 24-hour food recall, the interviewer asks the patient to recall everything he or she ate and drank for the previous day. For persons working odd hours or eating at night, it is important to include a complete 24-hour period starting at 12:00 A.M. To help the patient remember what was eaten and drunk, ask what he or she did that day. For instance, the beginning of a 24-hour recall interview might proceed as follows:

> "About what time did you get up yesterday? And what was the first thing you ate or drank? Then what did you do? Did you eat or drink anything then?"

Some patients might have an easier time remembering what they ate and drank from the most recent meal backwards:

> "Did you eat or drink anything in the middle of the night last night? Did you have anything before you went to bed? What did you have for supper?"

The interviewer must remember to ask specific questions about portion size; how food was prepared; and whether toppings such as butter, margarine, or dressing were added at the table. Food models can often assist patients in estimating portion size.

Twenty-four hour recalls are fairly quick, inexpensive, and do not require a high level of patient effort. Interactive computerized 24-hour recall programs are also available. However, food intake in one 24-hour period may not give a true representation of usual food intake. For more accurate estimates of usual intake, several recalls are needed. Some patients may have trouble remembering what they ate the previous day, hence, underestimating food intake. Also, some individuals tend to tailor recall to what they think the interviewer expects to hear.

Food Frequency Questionnaires

Questionnaires that ask how frequently the patient consumes certain foods can also give insight into dietary habits of obese persons. Food frequency questionnaires are quick and easy to complete and provide insight on consumption of certain types of high-calorie or high-fat foods. However, food frequency questionnaires do not provide very accurate information on quantity.

Following is a sample questionnaire that combines weight history and lifestyle habits with food frequency questions:

1. What has been your heaviest weight?

2. How much did you weigh at the following ages: birth, age 10, age 15, age 25, and now?

3. Describe the following members of your family as thin, average, heavy, or obese: your spouse, yourself, your mother, your father, your sisters, your brothers, your own children.

4. How do you spend a typical day? Ask the patient to elaborate, for example, reading, studying, watching television (remember the earlier figures about the average child spending nearly 23 hours a week in front of the television?), or physical activities, such as aerobics,

jogging, or traveling.

5. What type of job do you have—how do you spend a typical day on the job?

6. Do you eat out often? How frequently?

7. Do you have any sleeping problems? How many hours do you sleep during an average night?

8. How much exercise do you get regularly? Are you less active than you once were?

9. What are your interests and hobbies?

10. Do you have long stretches of time with nothing to do? If so, can you explain why?

11. What are the reasons you want to lose weight?

12. Why do you think you are overweight?

13. How much do you want to lose, and what do you think is your goal weight?

14. Have you ever devised a diet of your own? Describe it, and how long you were on it.

15. How many times have you tried to lose weight in the past? What ways did you use? Did they work, or did you regain your lost weight?

16. When do you usually eat your meals? Breakfast? Lunch? Dinner?

17. Do you eat vegetables every day? Fruits?

18. Do you eat cereals and whole grains?

19. Do you drink milk or eat dairy products? How often?

20. How many cups of coffee and/or tea do you drink every day?

21. Do you drink soft drinks, and, if so, how many per day?

22. Do you drink alcoholic beverages? How much? How often?

23. Estimate your total fluid intake per day. Would you estimate this to be 1 quart? 2 quarts? Less?

24. Do you ever estimate your daily caloric intake, and can you do it correctly? If so, what is the average day's total calories for you?

25. Are there types of foods you like better than others; are there types you dislike more than others?

26. How many meals per day do you eat?

27. How often do you eat snacks?

28. What do you eat during snack time?

29. What makes you choose the foods you do? Environment? Hunger? Stress? Taste, sight of

---

TABLE 5.7 Laboratory Assessment of Medical Conditions Associated with Obesity

If suspicion of...	*Consider...*
Cushing's syndrome	24-hour urine collection to be tested for free cortisol (>150 micrograms/24 hours; abnormal), plus low-dose dexamethasone suppression test of 0.5 milligrams every 6 hours for 2 days, with collection of 24-hour urine to test for 17-hydroxycorticosteroid levels on second day (>3.5 milligrams/24 hours; abnormal)
Hypothyroidism	Serum TSH level (normal, generally <5 microunits/milliliter)
Diabetes	Fasting serum glucose level
Hyperlipidemia	Fasting total levels of cholesterol, triglycerides, HDL cholesterol
Gallstones	Ultrasonography
Periodic/sleep apnea	Sleep studies for oxygen desaturation; ENT exam for upper airway obstruction

Note: TSH, thyroid-stimulating hormone; HDL, high-density lipoprotein; ENT ear, nose, and throat.

Source: Weinsier, R. L (1995). Clinical assessment of obese patients. In K. D. Brownell, & C. G. Fairburn, (Eds.). *Eating disorders and obesity,* (pp. 463–468). New York: The Guilford Press.

food, craving for a certain food? Social pressure? Time pressure? Travel? Ethnic or cultural conditioning? Habit?

30. Do you have specific associations with certain foods? (That is, do certain foods evoke emotions or association with persons or places?)

LABORATORY STUDIES

Routine laboratory assessment of patients with obesity and eating disorders includes

- Complete blood count (CBC)

- Electrolytes

- Blood urea nitrogen (BUN)

- Creatinine

For patients with eating disorders, an EKG may be done if there has been significant weight loss, hypokalemia, or abuse of syrup of ipecac. Liver enzymes should be checked in patients with rapid weight loss or in those suspected of abusing alcohol, since liver damage can result from wasting of the liver and fat deposition. Patients with gastrointestinal bleeding should have their stool examined for blood. Serum calcium and phosphate levels should also be assessed in patients who are emaciated or have chronic amenorrhea (Kaplan and Garfinkle, 1993).

For the obese patient, laboratory tests should be based on findings of the physical examination. *Table 5.7* suggests specific laboratory tests based on medical findings.

The next chapter describes treatment goals, factors to consider, and types of approaches for management of both obesity and eating disorders.

EXAM QUESTIONS

CHAPTER 5
Questions 34–39

34. Which of the following are elements of a baseline health history for a patient who is obese or has an eating disorder?

    a. questions on past weight control treatments and responses

    b. body mass index

    c. food frequency records

    d. complete blood count

35. About what percentage of patients with anorexia nervosa vomit regularly?

    a. 5 percent

    b. 10 percent

    c. 25 percent

    d. 50 percent

36. Which of the following instruments is considered a "gold standard" for the assessment of eating disorders?

    a. The Eating Disorders Assessment Scale

    b. The Eating Disorders Examination

    c. The Borderline Personality Disorder Inventory

    d. The Minnesota Multi Phasic Inventory

37. Which of the following is used to assess distribution of body fat?

    a. relative weight

    b. body mass index

    c. waist-to-hip ratio

    d. mean upper arm circumference

38. Keeping a daily 24-hour food intake record is most useful in dietary assessment of individuals with obesity or eating because

    a. it provides a comparison of food intake over time.

    b. it helps the patient become aware of his or her own food behavior.

    c. it permits precise calorie measurements.

    d. it documents noncompliance with the diet.

39. Routine laboratory assessment of patients with obesity and eating disorders includes which of the following?

    a. electrolytes

    b. electrocardiogram

    c. serum calcium and phosphate levels

    d. liver enzymes

CHAPTER 6

PLANNING: MATCHING PATIENTS AND TREATMENTS

CHAPTER OBJECTIVE

After reading this chapter, you will be able to indicate appropriate therapy options for patients with varying degrees of obesity, eating disorders, and medical risk.

LEARNING OBJECTIVES

After studying this chapter, you will be able to

1. Recognize goals for the treatment of obesity and eating disorders.

2. Specify factors to consider when planning intervention for patients with obesity or eating disorders.

3. Differentiate between different types of treatments for obesity or eating disorders.

4. Select appropriate treatment options for a variety of patients with obesity or eating disorders.

INTRODUCTION

After a thorough initial assessment, the nurse and other health professionals must work with the patient to plan an appropriate course of therapy. Because each patient is unique and because so many factors contribute to weight disturbances, there are numerous approaches to management of both obesity and eating disorders. No one approach works for everyone.

According to Robison (1993), elements of a successful weight-management program

1. Are individualized to the needs and medical status of the patient

2. Are multidisciplinary in nature, involving trained practitioners from medicine, psychology, nutrition and exercise physiology all working with the patient as a team

3. Are long-term, with on-going intervention and support even after weight loss or stabilization has been achieved

4. Address psychological and social barriers to lifetime weight control

5. Encourage family and peer support

6. Foster positive self-image and better quality of life

Regardless of the means to accomplish weight loss, stabilization, or nutritional repletion, weight-management interventions should emphasize lifetime changes in diet, exercise, behavior, and attitudes to promote permanent weight control.

PLANNING INTERVENTIONS FOR OBESE PATIENTS

Treatment Goals

Setting realistic goals is a critical element of successful weight loss interventions. Willard (1991) stated, "weight-loss by itself is not a worthwhile treatment goal, because weight is often regained." Rather, maintenance of weight loss must be the ultimate goal of any obesity intervention program. Weight loss requires only a short-term energy deficit. Weight control, however, requires lifelong behavior changes.

Achieving this ultimate goal requires setting a series of short-term goals, including goals for weight loss. The need for weight loss should be driven by medical considerations, not cosmetic ones. Based on a national consensus conference on obesity (National Institutes of Health, 1985), weight loss is recommended for persons exceeding desirable weight by 20 percent or more. For individuals with type II diabetes, high blood pressure, or high blood lipid levels, weight reduction may be helpful at lesser degrees of overweight.

Many patients need not, and probably should not, aim for desirable body weight according to height/weight tables as a short-term goal weight (Blackburn, 1987). Setting unrealistically high goals can be mentally and physically self-defeating.

In a position paper on weight control, The American Dietetic Association (1989) states:

"...optimal weight is the most favorable weight for an individual as determined by a variety of factors, such as existing health problems (hypertension, diabetes, heart disease), percentage of body fat, location of excess fat in the body, age, sex, heredity, psychological implications, and realistic weight maintenance goals. For some persons, optimal weight will be more or less

than the weight allowed by accepted weight-for-height tables."

Well-known obesity expert Dr. George Blackburn suggests setting a short-term weight-loss goal of 10 to 15 percent of current body weight for any single treatment course, which would last six months to one year. A loss of 10 to 15 percent of body weight improves heart function, blood pressure, glucose tolerance and many other medical conditions in 9 out of 10 patients. According to Blackburn, after this weight loss has been maintained for a year or more, the patient can strive to reduce body weight another 10 to 15 percent toward a long-term goal of a BMI of less than 30.

Successful outcomes of weight-loss programs can be interpreted many ways. In its landmark report, *Weighing the Options: Criteria for Evaluating Weight Management Programs,* the Food and Nutrition Board (1995) give four measures of successful weight management programs:

1. **Long-Term Weight Loss** Successful programs yield a loss of >5 percent of body weight or a reduction in BMI of 1 unit or more over one year or more.

2. **Improvement in Obesity-Related Health Problems** Successful programs should improve obesity-related health problems such as high blood pressure, high blood lipid levels, or type II diabetes, if present.

3. **Improved Health Practices** Successful programs foster improved health practices such as good eating habits, regular physical activity, obtaining regular medical care, and screening and follow-up for obesity-related health problems.

Factors to Consider

Many factors affect selection of an appropriate weight-loss program, including those related to the individual and those related to the specific program (Food and Nutrition Board, 1995). Factors relating to the individual include

- Degree of obesity

- Personal weight-loss goals

- Age

- Level of motivation

- Readiness to change

- Health status

- Weight-related risk factors

- Influence of family, friends, health-care providers, and the media

- The individual's assessment of the need for outside help

Factors relating to the program include

- Availability and cost of a program

- Intensity of the program

- Nature, or type, of program

- The soundness and safety of the program

- Evidence of successful outcomes of the program

Table 6.1 shows guidelines for sound weight-management programs developed by the Task Force to Establish Weight Loss Guidelines for Michigan (1990).

Types of Therapies

Approaches to weight loss range from conservative to aggressive, and from self-directed to those with intensive medical monitoring. The literally hundreds of weight-management approaches can be broadly classified into three categories (Food and Nutrition Board, 1995):

- Do-it-yourself programs

- Nonclinical programs

- Clinical programs

Do-it-yourself programs are a plan of weight loss that the individual formulates and directs by hisself or herself. Individuals may use guidance from a popular diet book, magazine, or self-help group such as TOPS (Take Off Pounds Sensibly) or

Overeaters Anonymous. Individuals may also use commercially available diet foods or meal replacements, but they do so without supervision.

Nonclinical programs are usually commercially franchised programs with parent companies providing guidance and materials to each franchise. Although the parent company usually employs health care professionals in developing materials, qualifications and training of counselors at each franchise can vary substantially. Examples of nonclinical programs include Diet Center, Jenny Craig, Nutri/System, and Weight Watchers.

Clinical weight-loss programs are directed and supervised by trained health care professionals, such as nurses, physicians, and dietitians. Clinical programs include individual counseling with a health care professional as well as multidisciplinary group programs. Examples of clinical programs include Health Management Resources (HMR), Medifast, New Direction, and Optifast. *Table 6.2* gives some background information on some of the more popular weight-loss programs.

Whether the weight-loss program is do-it-yourself, nonclinical, or clinical, each uses one or more of the following approaches

- Diet

- Physical activity

- Behavior modification

- Drug therapy

- Gastric surgery

More information on each of these approaches will be given in chapters seven through nine, but they will also be reviewed briefly below.

Diet

Dietary changes for weight loss can be grouped into three categories based on calorie level.

Balanced deficit diets provide at least 1,200 calories daily and are usually nutritionally adequate if the diet is varied and includes at least the mini-

---

TABLE 6.1 Recommendations for Adult Weight Loss Programs

Screening: The client should be screened, and the level of health risk should be identified: low, moderate, or high.

Individualized treatment plan: Factors contributing to the client's weight status should be identified. These factors should determine the relative importance of diet, exercise, behavioral change, medical monitoring or supervision, and health supervision in each individualized treatment plan.

Staffing: Weight loss service providers should be trained and appropriately supervised for each level of health risk of clients receiving care.

Full disclosure: The client should give informed consent, having been informed of any potential physical and psychological risks of weight loss, the probable long-term success of the program, the full cost of the program, and the professional credentials of the service providers.

Reasonable weight goal: The weight goal for the client should be based on personal and family history and not exclusively on height and weight charts.

Rate of weight loss: The advertised and actual rate of weight loss, after the first 2 weeks, should not exceed an average of 2 pounds per week.

Calories per day: The daily caloric intake should not be lower than 1,000 kilocalories without medical supervision. If the daily caloric intake is below 800 kilocalories, additional safeguards should be in place. Even with medical supervision, 600 kilocalories per day is the lowest recommended intake.

Diet composition
- **Protein:** between 0.8 and 1.5 grams protein per kilogram of goal body weight, but no more than 100 grams protein per day.
- **Fat:** 10% to 30% of energy as fat.
- **Carbohydrate:** at least 100 grams per day without medical supervision; at least 50 grams per day even with medical supervision.
- **Fluid:** at least 1 quart water daily.

Nutritional adequacy: The food plan should allow the client to obtain 100% of the Recommended Dietary Allowances (RDAs). If nutritional supplements are used, nutrient levels should not greatly exceed 100% of the RDA.

Nutrition education: Nutrition education encouraging permanent healthful eating patterns should be incorporated into the weight loss program.

Formula products: The food plan should consist of foods available from the conventional food supply. Formula products are not recommended for the treatment of moderate obesity and should not be used at low-calorie formulations without specialized medical supervision.

Exercise component: The weight loss program should include an exercise component that is safe and appropriate for the individual client:
- The client should be screened for conditions that would require medical clearance before starting an exercise program.
- The client should be instructed on how to recognize and deal with potentially dangerous physical responses to exercise.
- The client should work toward 30 to 60 minutes of continuous exercise five to seven times per week, with gradual increases in intensity and duration.

Psychological Component: Appropriate behavior modification techniques should be incorporated into the individualized weight loss program.

Appetite suppressants: Appetite suppressant drugs are not recommended and should not take the place of changes in diet, exercise, and behavior.

Weight maintenance: A maintenance phase should be included. Programs should place as high a priority on helping clients maintain weight loss as on achieving initial weight loss.

Source: Task Force to Establish Weight Loss Guidelines for Michigan. (1990). *Toward safe weight loss: recommendations for adult weight loss programs in Michigan.* East Lansing, MI: Michigan Health Council.

---

mum servings recommended from all food groups. Unless the individual has other health problems, medical supervision is not required for balanced deficit diets.

Contrary to the beliefs of some patients, most individuals will lose weight on 1,200 calories daily. Lichtman and colleagues (1992) studied individuals who believed they failed to lose weight on less than 1,200 calories daily by evaluating total energy intake and actual energy expenditure in a metabolic

TABLE 6.2 Background Information on Some Popular Weight Loss Programs

DO-IT-YOURSELF PROGRAMS

Overeaters Anonymous (OA)

Approach/Method
Nonprofit international organization that provides volunteer support groups worldwide patterned after the 12-step Alcoholics Anonymous program. Addresses physical, emotional, and spiritual recovery aspects of compulsive overeating. Members encouraged to seek professional help for individualized diet/nutrition plan and for any emotional or physical problems.

Clients
Individuals who define themselves as compulsive eaters.

Staff
Nonprofessional volunteer group members who meet specific criteria lead meetings, sit on the board, and conduct activities.

Expected Weight Loss/Length of Program
Makes no claims for weight loss. Unlimited length.

Cost
Self-supporting with member contributions and sales of publications (includes workbooks, tapes, newsletters, and sponsor outreach programs). Its international monthly journal, *Lifeline,* costs $12.99/year.

Healthy Lifestyle Components
Recommends emotional, spiritual, and physical recovery changes. Makes no exercise or food recommendations.

Comments
Inexpensive. Provides group support. No need to follow a specific diet plan to participate. Minimal organization at the group level, so groups vary in approach. No health-care providers on staff.

Availability
10,500 groups in 47 countries. Headquarters: Rio Rancho, NM (505) 891-2664.

TOPS (Take Off Pounds Sensibly)

Approach/Method
Nonprofit support organization of 310,000 members who meet weekly in groups. Does not prescribe or endorse particular eating or exercise regimen. Mandatory weigh-in at weekly meetings. Provides peer support. Uses award programs for healthy lifestyle changes; special recognition given to best weight losers. Members who maintain their goal weight loss for 3 months become members of KOPS (Keep Off Pounds Sensibly).

Clients
Members must submit weight goals and diets obtained from a health professional in writing.

Staff
Each group elects a volunteer (non-health professional) to direct and organize activities for one year. Health professionals, including R.D.s and psychologists, may be invited to speak at weekly meetings. Organization consults with a medical advisor.

Expected Weight Loss/Length of Program
No claims made for weight loss. Unlimited length.

Cost
First visit free. $16 annual fee ($20 in Canada) for the first 2 years; $14 annually thereafter ($18 in Canada). Includes 40-page quarterly magazine from company headquarters. Weekly meetings cost 50 cents to $1.

Healthy Lifestyle Components
No official lifestyle or exercise recommendations, but endorses slow, permanent lifestyle changes. Members encouraged to consult health-care provider for an exercise regimen to meet their needs.

Comments
Inexpensive form of continuing group support. Used as adjunct to professional care. Nonprofit and noncommercial, so no purchases required. Encourages long-term participation. Lacks professional guidance at chapter level since meetings run by volunteers. Groups vary widely in approach.

Availability
11,700 chapters in 20 countries, mostly U.S. and Canada. Headquarters: Milwaukee, WI (800) 932-8677.

NONCLINICAL PROGRAMS

Diet Center

Approach/Method
Focuses on achieving healthy body composition through diet and personalized exercise recommendations under the name *Exclusively You Weight Management Program.* Diet based on regular supermarket food; Diet Center prepackaged cuisine is optional. Body-fat analysis via electrical impedance taken at start of program and every 4 to 6 weeks thereafter. Clients encouraged to visit center daily for weigh-in. Calorie levels individualized to meet client needs and goals. Minimum level: 1,200 kcal/day. Four phases: 2-day conditioning phase prepares dieter for reducing. Reducing phase used until goal achieved. Stabilization, the third phase, has clients adjusting calories and physical activity to maintain weight. Maintenance, the fourth phase, lasts for 1 year. One-to-one counseling. Some group meetings available.

Clients
Not allowed to join: pregnant, lactating, anorectic, bulimic, and underweight individuals, and those under 18 years of age. Require physician's written approval: those with more than 50 pounds to lose, kidney or heart disease, diabetes, cancer, or emphysema.

Staff
Clients consult with nonprofessional counselors who typically are program graduates trained by Diet Center. Two staff R.D.s and scientific advisors made up of a variety of health professionals design program at corporate level.

Expected Weight Loss/Length of Program
Not more than 1.5 to 2 pounds weekly. Length will vary with individualized client goals, but 1-year maintenance program strongly encouraged.

TABLE 6.2 Background Information on Some Popular Weight Loss Programs *(Cont.)*

Cost
Varies. Ranges from about $35 to $50/week. The 1-year maintenance is a one-time flat fee ranging from $50 to $200. Some centers charge additional one-time fee for all body composition analyses and adjustments in diet and exercise goals.

Healthy Lifestyle Components
Exclusively Me behavior management, as an ongoing part of the program, includes an activity book, audio tapes, and counseling. Used in conjunction with regular one-to-one sessions; counselor helps client design personal solutions to weight-control problems.

Comments
Emphasizes body composition, not pounds, as a measure of health. Does not require the purchase of Diet Center food for participation. Professional guidance lacking at the client level. Little group support available. Vitamin supplement required.

Availability
700 centers in U.S., Canada, Bermuda, Guam, and South America. Headquarters: Pittsburgh, PA (800) 333-2581.

Jenny Craig

Approach/Method
Personal Weight Management menu plans based on Jenny Craig's cuisine with additional store-bought foods. Diet ranges from 1,000 to 2,600 kcal, depending on client needs. Mandatory weekly one-to-one counseling; group workshops. After clients lose half their goal, they begin planning their own meals using their own foods.

Clients
Not allowed to join: individuals who are underweight, pregnant, or those below age 13; those with celiac disease, diabetes (who inject more than twice daily or who are under 18 years of age), or allergies to ubiquitous ingredients in company's food products. Require physician's written permission: individuals with 18 additional conditions. Regardless of condition, clients encouraged to communicate with personal physician throughout program.

Staff
Program developed by corporate R.D.s and psychologists. Company consults with advisory board of M.D.s, R.D.s, and Ph.D.s on program design. Consultants trained by Jenny Craig to implement program and offer support and motivational strategies. Corporate dietitians available for client questions or concerns at no extra charge.

Expected Weight Loss/Length of Program
Clients encouraged to set reasonable weight goals based on personal history and healthy weight standards. Program designed to produce weight loss of 1 to 2 pounds/week. A separate, 12-month maintenance program is also offered.

Cost
To join: $99 to $299, depending on option. Prices vary per inclusion of home audio and videocassettes. Most

expensive price includes *Lifestyle Maintenance* program. Jenny Craig cuisine costs average $70 weekly.

Healthy Lifestyle Components
Clients use program guides to learn cognitive behavioral techniques for relapse prevention and problem management for lifestyle changes. Based on individual priorities, clients address major factors involved with weight management (e.g., exercise, which is addressed through a physical activity module and a walking program). Individual consultations; group workshops provide motivation and peer exchange *The Lifestyle Maintenance* program addresses issues such as body image and maintaining motivation to exercise.

Comments
Little food preparation. Vegetarian and kosher meal plans available; also plans for diabetic, hypoglycemic, and breastfeeding clients. Recipes provided. Must rely on Jenny Craig cuisine for participation. Lack of professional guidance at client level.

Availability
800 centers in five countries; 650 centers in U.S. Headquarters: Del Mar, CA (800) 94-JENNY.

Nutri/System

Approach/Method
Menu plans based on Nutri/System's prepared meals with additional grocery foods. Clients receive individual calorie levels ranging from 1,000 to 2,200 kcal/day. Multivitamin-mineral supplement available for clients. Personal counseling and group sessions available.

Clients
Not allowed to join: individuals who are pregnant, under 14 years of age, underweight, or anorectic. Require physician's written permission: lactating women and those with a variety of conditions including diabetes (if require insulin shots), heart disease (that limits normal activity), and kidney disease.

Staff
Staff dietitians, health educators, and Ph.D.s develop program at corporate level. Scientific Advisory Board consisting of M.D.s and Ph.D.s employed for program design. Counselors with education and experience in psychology, nutrition, counseling, and health-related fields provide weekly guidance to clients. Certified Personal Trainers administer the Personal Trainer Program developed in conjunction with Johnson & Johnson Advanced Behavioral Technologies, Inc. R.D.s available through a toll-free number to address client questions.

Expected Weight Loss/Length of Program
Averages 1.5 to 2 pounds/week. Clients select weight goal based on a recommended weight range using standard tables. Program length varies with weight-loss goals.

Cost
Varies. Clients can lose all desired weight for $99.

TABLE 6.2 Background Information on Some Popular Weight Loss Programs *(Cont.)*

Unlimited service program costs $249. Food costs average $49/week. Vitamin-mineral supplements, at-home cholesterol test, motivational audiotapes, and exercise audio/videocassettes available at additional cost.

Healthy Lifestyle Components

Wellness and Personal Trainer services developed in conjunction with Johnson & Johnson Health Management have been added to the program.

Comments

Few decisions about what to eat; relatively rigid diet with company foods. Portion-controlled Nutri/System foods allow dieters to focus more on making lifestyle changes than on the reducing diet. Program provides both Wellness and Personal Trainer services. Little contact with health professionals.

Availability

650 centers in U.S. and Canada. Headquarters: Horsham, PA (215) 442-5411.

Weight Watchers

Approach/Method

Emphasis on portion control and healthy lifestyle habits. Dieters choose from regular supermarket food, *Weight Watchers Personal Cuisine* (available in select markets to members only), or both. Reducing phase: Women average 1,250 kcal daily; men, 1,600 daily. Levels for weight maintenance determined individually. Weekly group meetings with mandatory weigh-in. Must need to lose at least 5 pounds to join.

Clients

Not allowed to join: those not weighing at least 5 pounds above the lowest end of their healthy weight range and those with a medically diagnosed eating disorder. Require physician's written approval: pregnant and lactating women and children under 10 years of age.

Staff

Group leaders are non-health professional graduates of program (Lifetime Members) trained by Weight Watchers. Program developed by corporate R.D.s. Company consults with medical advisor and advisory board consisting of M.D.s and Ph.D.s on program design. Health professionals at corporate level, including R.D.s, direct program.

Expected Weight Loss/Length of Program

Up to 2 pounds weekly. Unlimited length. Special 2-week Superstart program offers more rapid initial weight loss. Maintenance plan is 6 weeks.

Cost

$17–$20 to join; $10–$13 weekly. Fee entitles member to unlimited meetings for that week. Monthly meetings are free for Lifetime Members who have completed maintenance plan and maintain their weight goal within 2 pounds. *Personal Cuisine* prices vary, averaging about $70 weekly.

Healthy Lifestyle Components

Emphasizes making positive lifestyle changes, including regular exercise. Encourages daily minimum physical activity level.

Comments

Flexible program offering group support and well-balanced diet. Vegetarian plan available, plus healthy eating plans for pregnant and breastfeeding women. Encourages long-term participation for members to attain their weight-loss goals. Lacks professional guidance at client level. No personalized counseling except in select markets.

Availability

29,000 weekly meetings in 24 countries. Headquarters: Jericho, NY (516) 939-0400.

CLINICAL PROGRAMS

Health Management Resources (HMR)

Approach/Method

Medically supervised very-low-calorie diet (VLCD) of fortified, high-protein liquid meal replacements (520 to 800 kcal daily) or a low-calorie option consisting of liquid supplements and prepackaged HMR entrees (800 to 1,300 kcal daily). Dieters receive HMR Risk Factor Profile that measures and displays an individual's medical and lifestyle health risks. Mandatory weekly 90-minute group meetings. Maintenance meetings are 1 hour per week. One-to-one counseling. Need to have BMI >30 for VLCD.

Clients

Contraindications: pregnancy, lactation, and acute substance abuse. Require physician's written approval: some with acute psychiatric disorders, recent heart disease, cancer, renal or liver disease, insulin-dependent diabetes mellitus, and those who test positive for acquired immunodeficiency syndrome (AIDS).

Staff

Program developed by M.D.s, R.D.s, R.N.s, and psychologists. Each location has at least one M.D. and health educator on staff. Participants assigned "personal coaches" (R.D.s, exercise physiologists, health educators) who help dieters learn and practice weight-management skills. Dieters on VLCD see M.D. or R.N. weekly.

Expected Weight Loss/Length of Program

Averages 2 to 5 pounds weekly. Reducing phase varies according to weight-loss needs, but averages 12 weeks; refeeding phase (after liquids only) lasts about 6 weeks. Maintenance program recommended for up to 18 months.

Cost

Varies depending on diet chosen and medical conditions. Ranges from $80 to $130/week including medical visits. Cost may be covered by insurance. Maintenance is $60–$90/month.

TABLE 6.2 Background Information on Some Popular Weight Loss Programs *(Cont.)*

Healthy Lifestyle Components

Recommends every client burn a minimum of 2,000 kcal in physical activity weekly. Advocates consuming a diet with no more than 30 percent of calories from fat and at least 35 servings of fruits and vegetables per week. Emphasizes lifestyle issues in weekly classes and in personal coaching.

Comments

Emphasizes exercise as a means for weight loss and control. Few decisions about what to eat. Supervised by a health professional. Requires a strong commitment to physical activity. Side effects of VLCD may include intolerance to cold, constipation, dizziness, dry skin, and headaches. All options include liquid supplement; diet is very high in protein, even at higher calorie levels.

Availability

180 hospitals and medical settings nationwide. Headquarters: Boston, MA (617) 357-9876.

Medifast

Approach/Method

Medifast is a physician-supervised very-low-calorie diet program of fortified meal replacements containing 450-500 kcal/day. *LifeStyles—The Medifast Program of Patient Support®* prepares patients to maintain their goal weight after completing the VLCD. Medifast also provides a low-calorie diet of approximately 860 kcal/day for those not indicated for the VLCD.

Clients

Contraindications: those who are not at least 30 percent above ideal body weight, those who have not reached sexual and physical maturation, pregnant and lactating women, those with a history of cerebrovascular accident, and those with conditions such as anorexia nervosa, bulimia, recent myocardial infarction, unstable angina, insulin-dependent diabetes, thrombophlebitis, active cancer, and uncompensated renal or hepatic disease.

Staff

Program supervised by a physician. At the corporate level, a medical advisory board of M.D.s, Ph.D.s, and R.D.s is consulted on program development.

Expected Weight Loss/Length of Program

Physician and patient arrive at an individualized goal weight. Metropolitan Life Insurance Company tables, Dietary Guidelines for Americans, and BMI charts used as guides. Weight loss varies with individual; average weight loss is 3-5 pounds/week. Weight Reduction Phase lasts 16 weeks and Realimentation Phase lasts 4–6 weeks. Maintenance strongly encouraged for up to 1 year.

Cost

Cost for office visits, laboratory tests, and Medifast products vary by individual physician. The program ranges from $65 to $85/week. Costs may be covered by insurance.

Healthy Lifestyle Components

The Medifast program includes a comprehensive education program called LifeStyles that includes behavior modification, recommended physical activity, and nutrition education. Instruction booklets and patient guides provided, including quarterly newsletter to patients.

Comments

Close contact with one or more health professionals. Low calorie level promotes quick weight loss. Extensive product line. Company products and regular foods incorporated when VLCD not recommended. Must rely on company products during reducing phase. Maintenance program assists with transition to regular foods.

Availability

15,000 physicians nationwide, primarily in office-based settings, and in six foreign countries. Headquarters: Jason Pharmaceuticals, Inc., Owings Mills, MD (410) 581-8042.

New Direction

Approach/Method

The New Direction System includes a medically supervised VLCD program of fortified meal replacements with 600-840 kcal/day. The OUTLook and ShapeWise programs are moderate-calorie programs of 1,000-1,500 kcal/day and include the use of regular food and fortified bars and beverages.

Clients

Contraindications to VLCD: women with less than 40 pounds to lose and men with less than 50 pounds to lose (except in special cases), those less than 18 years of age, pregnant and lactating women, and those with conditions such as insulin-dependent (type I) diabetes, metastatic cancer, recent myocardial infarction, liver disease requiring protein restriction, and renal insufficiency.

Staff

Weekly sessions in the New Direction and OUTLook programs are led by health professionals with degrees in dietetics, exercise physiology, behavioral counseling, or related fields. One-on-one counseling in each discipline is part of the program. Each program has a medical director.

Expected Weight Loss/Length of Program

In the New Direction program, average weight losses of 3 pounds/week after the first few weeks are common. In the OUTLook and ShapeWise programs, losses greater than 2 pounds/week are grounds for concern (after the first 2 weeks). The Reducing Phase averages 12–16 weeks, the Adapting Phase (with transition to regular food) lasts 5 weeks, and the Sustaining Phase is a minimum of 6 months (12 months preferred). Ongoing continuing care is encouraged.

Cost

Varies with the program chosen, amount of weight to

TABLE 6.2 Background Information on Some Popular Weight Loss Programs *(Cont.)*

lose, and medical conditions. An approximate range is $40/week in the OUTLook and ShapeWise programs; $110–$120/week in the Reducing Phase of the VLCD and $0-$20/week in the later phases. Costs may be covered by insurance.

Healthy Lifestyle Components

Weekly classes have a strong behavioral component with an emphasis on problem-solving and lifestyle-skills development in nutrition and exercise.

Comments

Individualized care and close contact with health professionals. Must rely on company products during the Reducing Phase of VLCD program. Transition from VLCD to regular food requires supervision. Low calorie level promotes quick weight loss, most beneficial for people with certain health problems. Clients make few decisions about what to eat while on the VLCD. OUTLook and ShapeWise programs include regular food.

Availability

Headquarters: Ross Products Division, Abbott Laboratories, Columbus, OH (614) 624-7573.

Optifast

Approach/Method

Medically supervised program of fortified liquid meal replacements and/or fortified food bars, eventually including more regular foods. Dieters assigned an 800-, 950-, or 1,200-kcal plan. Weekly sessions on how to change eating behavior and one-to-one counseling.

Clients

Not allowed to join: individuals less than 30 percent or less than 50 pounds over desirable weight (corresponding to a BMI of approximately 30-32) and those less than 18 years of age. Contraindications for the low-calorie protocol include pregnant and lactating women and individuals with recent acute myocardial infarction or unstable angina, insulin-dependent (type I) diabetes mellitus, and advanced liver or kidney disease.

Staff

Dieters seen regularly by M.D.s, R.N.s, R.D.s, and psychologists at most locations; exercise physiologist used on consulting basis. Group meeting leaders are psychologists or dietitians. Meetings often include R.D.s. Clients assigned case manager who coordinates care.

Expected Weight Loss/Length of Program

Program limits weight loss to 2 percent of body weight weekly. *Active Weight Loss Plan* lasts for about 13 weeks. Transition phase lasts for about 6 weeks. Maintenance, which begins at 20th week, is encouraged. No time limit on maintenance.

Cost

Varies with type of diet and length of program. Costs

range from $1,500 to $3,000, depending on health status and the amount of weight to lose. Price may include maintenance at some centers. Insurance may cover a portion of cost.

Healthy Lifestyle Components

Emphasis on behavior modification and diet planning for "real food" in group and counseling sessions. Exercise physiologist available to help design personal exercise plan.

Comments

Close contact with health professionals. Controlled calorie level promotes quick weight loss, most beneficial for people with certain health problems. Clients make few decisions about what to eat. Must rely on Optifast products during reducing phase.

Availability

Numerous hospitals and clinics in U.S. and foreign countries. Headquarters: Sandoz Nutrition, Minneapolis, MN (800) 662-2540.

Physicians in a Multidisciplinary Program

Approach/Method

Multidisciplinary programs may provide a program similar to HMR, New Direction, or Optifast. They may also provide food-based weight-loss programs or modifications of the two approaches. The multidisciplinary aspect implies the coordination of services, the availability of individual and/or group counseling, and comprehensive medical care.

Staff

Typically physicians, dietitians, behavior therapists, exercise physiologists, psychologists, and counselors working individually and in group settings. Service providers should be licensed and regulated and should have their activities scrutinized by peers.

Expected Weight Loss/Length of Program

Variable and adapted to the needs of patient. There should be a maintenance program with continuing patient access to services for sustaining care and reinforcement. Patient use of medications and consequences of surgery will be monitored.

Cost

Varies with approach used and duration. Some programs will use a standard professional fee-for-service schedule of charges; others will use a single charge for a comprehensive set of services for a specified period of time. Potential for reimbursement from health-insurance plans. A packaged set of services may be substantially less expensive than the individual services in a fee-for-service arrangement.

Health Lifestyle Components

Varies. All recognized factors in weight management will be considered.

TABLE 6.2 Background Information on Some Popular Weight Loss Programs *(Cont.)*

Comments

Similar to, but more extensive, services than physicians working alone. Professional staff coordinates all aspects of care and long-term management of obesity. Diverse staff is able to adapt care to the needs of patients, including the management of associated medical problems. These are often university-based programs, which have structured peer-review mechanisms and may conduct research. Costs for professional services tend to be high.

Availability

Very limited.

OTHERS

Registered Dietitians (R.D.s)

Approach/Method

Highly personalized approach to weight loss and maintenance.

Clients

Those acceptable and not acceptable will vary with the R.D.

Staff

R.D.s have, at a minimum, baccalaureate degrees in nutrition or closely related field and have completed approved or accredited clinical training. Often have advanced degrees. R.D.s must pass a registration examination given by the Commission on Dietetic Registration of the American Dietetic Association and participate in continuing education.

Expected Weight Loss/Length of Program

Varies according to weight goal. Clients rarely encouraged to lose more than 2 pounds weekly.

Cost

Varies across the country, but can range from $35 to $150 per hour. Fees for weight-control groups may be substantially less than for individual counseling.

Healthy Lifestyle Components

Exercise encouraged as part of safe, sensible weight-control program. R.D.s help clients identify barriers to weight loss and maintenance, and provide education about healthy lifestyles.

Comments

Highly adaptable. Personalized approach to clients' health concerns. Trained health professionals who can address medical history and account for it in diet therapy, if necessary. Appropriate for any age group. Can be expensive.

Availability

Located in every state in private practice, outpatient hospital clinics, health maintenance organizations (HMOs), and in practice with M.D.s. For a free referral to a local R.D., call (800) 366-1655.

Physicians Practicing Alone

Approach/Method

Individualized approach to weight loss and maintenance. Patients able to coordinate the management of their weight with concurrent management of associated medical problems. Services can be adapted to specific needs. Options include medications and surgery to treat obesity.

Staff

Individual physicians possibly working with associates (e.g., nurses and physicians' assistants). Provision of services by licensed professional health-care providers.

Expected weight Loss/Length of Program

Varies with patient. Program may be of indefinite length and should be coordinated with care of related or unrelated medical issues.

Cost

Varies. Fees will be comparable to those charged for comparable medical services. Cost may be reduced by reimbursement from health-insurance companies and avoidance of duplication of services in referrals for medical care by nonprofessional programs.

Healthy Lifestyle Components

Varies with the physician and weight-loss approach. Should include exercise and nutrition counseling.

Comments

Professional care. Coordination with other medical problems. Appropriate for patients with complex or serious associated medical problems. Long-term attention in the context of other medical care can be provided. The potential for using medications and/or surgery expands the opportunities for patients at varying stages of their disease. Individual physicians have the ability to vary the patient's care and intensity of the effort depending on the patient's life circumstances. Physicians often inadequately trained in nutrition and in low-calorie physiology. Cost for services can be high.

Availability

Generally available, but many physicians are reluctant to treat obesity because of their lack of interest or training, recognition that support services that they cannot provide are needed, and concern for the limited usefulness of their intervention.

SOURCE: Ward, E. M. (1994). Winners or losers? EN reviews the top weight-loss programs. *Environmental Nutrition.* 17:1, 3–5.

ward. In these individuals, failure to lose weight while dieting was due to underreporting of calorie intake and overestimation of physical activity.

Low-calorie diets provide 800 to 1,200 calories daily. Some of these diets use regular foods, while others use specially formulated foods or products. If the individual is following a low-calorie diet made up of regular foods, a vitamin and mineral supplement is probably needed.

Low-calorie diets are more appropriate for patients with obesity-related health problems. Patients using low-calorie diets should do so only after checking with their doctor and only under supervision by a health care provider. Often levels of blood pressure or diabetes medications need to be adjusted.

Very low-calorie diets (VLCD) are modified fasts, providing less than 800 calories daily. Most VLCD programs are specially prepared formula diets providing 0.8 to 1.5 grams of high-quality proteins per kilogram of body weight, up to 100 grams of carbohydrates, a minimum of essential fatty acids, the recommended allowances of vitamins and minerals, and electrolytes daily. Some VLCD use a combination of food and supplements. Most are used under intensive medical supervision and include a multidisciplinary education component taught by physicians, nurses, behavioral therapists, dietitians, and exercise physiologists.

VLCD are usually only appropriate for moderately or severely obese individuals with a BMI greater than 30 who have already tried more conservative weight-loss approaches. VLCD may also be appropriate for individuals with a BMI of 27 to 30 who have obesity-related health problems (Kanders and Blackburn, 1993).

Physical Activity

Physical activity should be a part of any weight-control program. Ample evidence indicates that regular physical activity increases weight loss in obese persons, especially when used in conjunction with dietary restriction (Bray, 1990; Fox, 1992). While weight losses from physical activity alone rarely exceed four to five pounds a month, over the long-term, such losses can be significant.

For weight control, the regularity of physical activity appears to be more important than the intensity, perhaps because of effects on appetite or metabolic rate (Willard, 1991). In addition, regular physical activity helps preserve lean body mass with weight loss. This means that a greater portion of the weight loss is from fat as opposed to muscle tissue. Low-intensity exercise appears to be just as effective as high-intensity exercise in preserving lean body mass (Ballor, 1990).

Regular physical activity is also one of the key ingredients in weight maintenance. According to a study by Van Dale and colleagues (1990), almost all subjects who maintained a regular exercise program were moderately successful in sustaining weight loss after 2 years. Over 70 percent of those who did not exercise regained 75 percent or more of their weight loss.

Besides its effects on body weight, inactivity is also an independent risk factor for coronary heart disease. Physical activity, with or without weight loss and dietary change reduces risk for coronary heart disease (Fox, 1992). Physical activity also improves lipid profiles, blood pressure, glucose tolerance, and enhances overall well-being.

Behavior Modification

Behavior modification was originally developed based on the theory that faulty eating behavior caused overeating and obesity. The goal of earlier programs was to restructure eating environment and eating behavior for permanent weight maintenance. However, weight losses on such programs were modest and weight maintenance was no better than with other interventions (Surgeon General's Report on Nutrition and Health, 1988).

Current behavior modification programs have

been broadened and now usually include a balanced low-calorie diet and exercise component. Such programs form the basis of many commercial weight loss regimens. Some behavior modification techniques can also be used in combination with other weight-loss therapies, such as very low-calorie diets.

Stunkard (1992) has summarized the key elements in five leading behavior modification manuals. These include

Stimulus Control—controlling food cues while grocery shopping, during activities, and at social events; preplanning and reordering eating environment.

Eating Behavior—putting utensils down in between bites, chewing slowly, preparing one portion at a time, avoiding other activities such as reading or watching television while eating.

Rewards—asking family and friends for encouragement, setting material rewards.

Self-Monitoring—keeping a food diary of time and place of eating, type and amount of food eaten, who was present, thought and feelings.

Nutrition Education—eating a healthy low-fat and high-carbohydrate diet, learning calorie values of foods.

Physical Activity—increasing routine activity throughout the day and beginning a regular aerobic exercise program.

Cognitive Restructuring—setting reasonable goals, thinking positive.

Drug Therapy

Interest in using drugs to help manage obesity has increased in recent years. The sentiment is that if physicians treat other chronic diseases with drugs over the long term, why can't they treat obesity with drugs over the long term? In a National Institutes of Health workshop on the pharmacological treatment of obesity, it was concluded that "obesity drugs produce short-term weight loss and remain effective in some patients" (Atkinson and Hubbard, 1994).

In April of 1996 the U.S. Food and Drug Administration approved dexfenfluramine, the first new antiobesity drug in 23 years. Meanwhile, physicians also increased prescriptions for a combination of two drugs—fenfluramine and phentermine, or fen-phen as the combination was nicknamed—that were each already approved by the FDA several years earlier but were never approved for combined use. Use of dexfenfluramine and the fen-phen combination skyrocketed over the next year and one-half, until research revealed potentially serious heart value damage in up to one-third of individuals who had used either drug alone or in combination with phentermine. In September of 1997, dexfenfluramine and fenfluramine were voluntarily withdrawn from the market by the manufacturers, although phentermine and other anti-obesity drugs are still available.

The health concerns and eventual recall of the two antiobesity drugs in 1997 highlight the fact that no simple cure for obesity exists. In all cases, risks of taking an antiobesity drug must be weighed against risks of remaining obese. Thus, drug therapy for obesity should be reserved for patients who are medically at risk and should be delivered as part of a comprehensive weight reduction program.

Gastric Surgery

Gastric surgery for obesity treatment should only be considered in patients who are severely obese (BMI of 40 or more, or BMI of 35 to 40 with co-existing medical problems) and have tried other weight-loss approaches. Candidates for surgery must be motivated, well-informed, and willing to participate in follow-up over the long-term.

Matching Approaches and Patients

As with other diseases, conservative therapies are usually tried before aggressive therapies. Conservative therapies for obesity treatment

TABLE 6.3 Obesity Management Options			
Degree of Obesity	*Percent over Desirable Weight*	*Body Mass Index*	*Options*
Mild	20–39%	27–30	conservative treatment
Moderate	40–100%	30–35	conservative treatment or very low-calorie diet
Severe	>100%	>35	very low-calorie diet or surgery

include a balanced deficit diet, exercise, and behavior change. More aggressive therapies may be appropriate when conservative treatment fails or when the degree of obesity or health risk warrant using them (Perri and colleagues, 1992).

Therapies can also be combined or undertaken in a stepped manner. For example, a phase of balanced low-calorie dieting plus behavior modification and exercise can follow a very low-calorie diet phase. All weight-loss interventions must teach sound nutrition, behavior change and exercise for long-term success.

Dr. Albert Stunkard (1992) of the University of Pennsylvania recommends considering obesity management options along the lines of obesity severity *(Table 6.3)*. Mild obesity, which affects about 90 percent of obese individuals, is usually best treated with conservative therapy unless there are medical indications for more aggressive treatment. Moderate obesity, which affects about 9 percent of obese individuals, can be treated with either conservative or aggressive therapy. Severe obesity, which affects less than 1 percent of obese individuals, is usually best treated with aggressive therapies such as surgery or very low-calorie diets.

Blackburn has developed a stepped-care model for obesity treatment *(Figure 6.1)* beginning with individual risk assessment and having as a goal preventing further weight gain or producing a weight loss of 2 BMI units (about 10 pounds). In this model, individual progress from conservative to aggressive weight-loss approaches based on their level of medical risk and outcomes of treatment. A similar model is illustrated in *Figure 6.2.*

FIGURE 6.1 Stepped-Care Model for Obesity Treatment

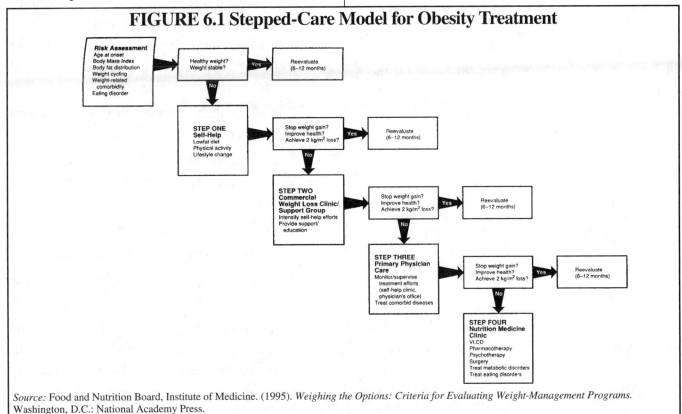

Source: Food and Nutrition Board, Institute of Medicine. (1995). *Weighing the Options: Criteria for Evaluating Weight-Management Programs.* Washington, D.C.: National Academy Press.

FIGURE 6.2 Three-Stage Process in Selecting a Weight Loss Program

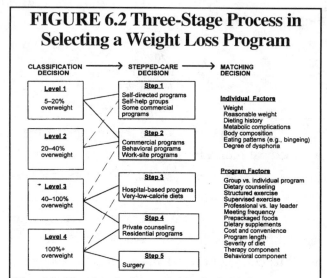

The classification decision divides individuals into four levels according to percentage of overweight. These levels dictate which of the five steps would be reasonable in the second stage, the stepped-care decision, on the principle that the least intensive, costly, and risky approach will be used from among alternative treatments. The third stage, the matching decision, is used to make the final selection of a program and is based on a combination of client and program variables. The dashed lines between the classification and stepped-care stages show the lowest level of treatment that may be beneficial, although more intensive treatment is usually necessary for people at the specified weight level.

Source: Adapted from Brownell and Wadden, 1991. Reprinted with permission of the Association for Advancement of Behavior Therapy.

Figure 6.3 illustrates the entire decision process in selecting a weight-loss program based on the match between the program and the consumer, the soundness and safety of the program, and the outcomes of the program.

PLANNING INTERVENTIONS FOR PATIENTS WITH EATING DISORDERS

Treatment Goals

Overall goals in treating individuals with eating disorders are to restore health and prevent relapse (Reichert, 1993). In striving to achieve these goals, the nurse will have to work with the patient on several levels simultaneously. Although treatment of eating disorders is most effective using a multidisciplinary team of health care professionals, the nurse is often the team member having the most contact and influence with the patient.

Patients with eating disorders have dysfunctional thoughts, attitudes, and behaviors relating to body image, relationships, and food. Although weight loss or erratic eating are symptoms of these dysfunctional beliefs, symptoms must be treated promptly to assure that the patient has adequate energy to tackle the underlying problems (Irwin, 1993).

Although psychological therapy and education is essential to treatment of patients with eating disorders, nutritional therapy to replete body weight or to stabilize erratic eating patterns is crucial to recovery and should be started immediately (Fichter, 1995). Patients will gain little from psychotherapy when they are starving or suffering from acute medical complications of eating disorders. Postponing discussion of nutritional therapy for individuals with eating disorders has been likened to postponing discussion of drinking behavior in treatment of alcoholic patients (Beaumont and Touyz, 1995).

Primary goals of nutrition therapy for patients with anorexia nervosa or bulimia nervosa are

- To achieve and maintain normal nutritional status in adults, or to attain and maintain normal growth in adolescents

- To establish normal eating behavior

- To promote a normal attitude toward food

- To promote normal responses to hunger and satiety cues (Beumont and Touyz, 1995)

As the patient begins to stabilize eating and pursue nutritional goals, the nurse and other members of the health care team can begin to assess and address underlying issues that contributed to devel-

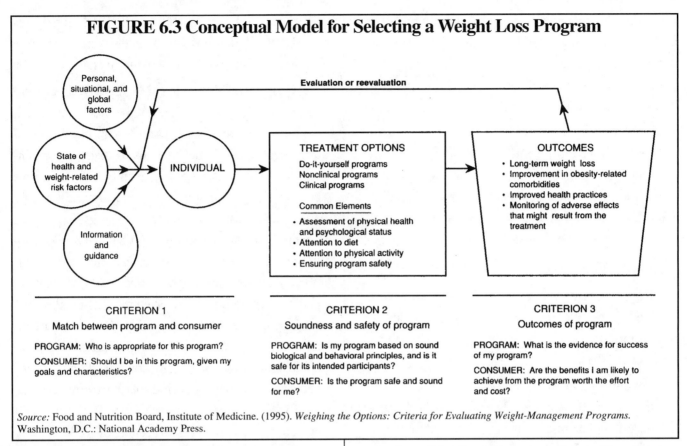

FIGURE 6.3 Conceptual Model for Selecting a Weight Loss Program

Personal, situational, and global factors

Evaluation or reevaluation

State of health and weight-related risk factors

INDIVIDUAL

Information and guidance

TREATMENT OPTIONS
Do-it-yourself programs
Nonclinical programs
Clinical programs

Common Elements
• Assessment of physical health and psychological status
• Attention to diet
• Attention to physical activity
• Ensuring program safety

OUTCOMES
• Long-term weight loss
• Improvement in obesity-related comorbidities
• Improved health practices
• Monitoring of adverse effects that might result from the treatment

CRITERION 1
Match between program and consumer

PROGRAM: Who is appropriate for this program?
CONSUMER: Should I be in this program, given my goals and characteristics?

CRITERION 2
Soundness and safety of program

PROGRAM: Is my program based on sound biological and behavioral principles, and is it safe for its intended participants?
CONSUMER: Is the program safe and sound for me?

CRITERION 3
Outcomes of program

PROGRAM: What is the evidence for success of my program?
CONSUMER: Are the benefits I am likely to achieve from the program worth the effort and cost?

Source: Food and Nutrition Board, Institute of Medicine. (1995). *Weighing the Options: Criteria for Evaluating Weight-Management Programs.* Washington, D.C.: National Academy Press.

opment of the eating disorder. Since the average recovery time for patients with eating disorders is five years or more, these issues need to be worked on over time. Long-term goals of therapy include modifying the patient's beliefs and attitudes about self, weight, and food. Nurses and therapists should address co-existing problems such as depression or anxiety. They should also explore the patient's relationship with the family or spouse and should involve these significant others in education and support.

Often achieving nutritional and long-term goals directly conflicts with what the patient desires. In inpatient treatment of patients with anorexia nervosa, for example, patients may hide food or refuse to eat. Nurses must strive to establish a trust relationship with the patient that includes establishing firm guidelines yet remaining empathetic to the patients' struggles.

Factors to Consider

Individuals with eating disorders have a broad variety of backgrounds, varying self-concepts, diverse beliefs and attitudes about food, and different levels of medical risk. All these factors must be considered in selecting a treatment approach for a patient with eating disorders.

Some patients are medically stable, while others are in acute medical danger. Some patients are fairly well-nourished, while others are emaciated. Patients with lower body weights and greater metabolic derangements need immediate and aggressive nutritional therapy to restore health and nutritional status. Although health risks are usually greater in patients with anorexia nervosa compared to patients with bulimia nervosa, potential risks for each patient must be individually assessed. The psychosocial well-being of patients must also be considered in planning a treatment approach. Many people with eating disorders have coexisting problems such as depression, low self-esteem, anxiety, obsessiveness, or personality disorders.

The patient's attitude toward treatment is also

important. Many patients deny they have a problem and resist treatment. Other patients have tried so many other treatments that they are either very discouraged or ready to try anything. Some patients believe they can recover on their own; others know they need help.

In planning family interventions, the need for education and functioning of the family unit must be considered. Since treatment of eating disorders often takes several years, financial resources of the patient must also be considered.

Types of Therapies

Regardless of the exact treatment approach selected, experts agree on five basic principles of management for patients with eating disorders (Fichter, 1995)

1. Psychological treatment or psychotherapy is the treatment of choice, but the type of therapy used is not as important as the individual therapist's own competence and experience in treating patients with eating disorders.

2. Weight gain and nutritional repletion should be an early goal so that the patient can gain the most benefit from psychotherapy.

3. Family, spouses, or significant others should be involved in the treatment process if possible.

4. Treatment should be individually designed to meet the patient's needs.

5. There should be as much continuity of care as possible.

Effective treatment programs for eating disorders are multidisciplinary, involving nurses, dietitians, physicians, psychologists or psychiatrists. Treatment can be done either on an inpatient or outpatient basis, with inpatient treatment usually reserved for patients at acute medical risk or for the purposes of brief, intensive education. Regardless of whether treatment is initiated in an inpatient or outpatient setting, long-term follow-up is usually needed, consisting of one or more of several possible approaches (Fairburn, 1995). Nutritional instruction and counseling is integral in all of these approaches and will be discussed in chapter ten.

Cognitive Behavioral Therapy Cognitive behavioral therapy is based on the view that certain cognitive characteristics interact with physiological and psychological mechanisms to foster and maintain the eating disorder. For example, the cognitive characteristic of judging self-worth by body weight and shape helps perpetuate an eating disorder. In cognitive behavior therapy, the therapist works with the patient to eliminate these dysfunctional cognitions. Treatment usually has three stages: (1) helping patients regain control over eating, (2) tackling the main precipitant of the eating disorder, and (3) maintaining changes and preventing relapse. Cognitive behavioral therapy is usually conducted on a one-to-one basis and over a period of four to five months and is considered the psychological treatment of choice for many patients with eating disorders.

Behavioral Therapy Behavioral therapy is most often used in combination with cognitive behavioral therapy. In behavior therapy, the patient is exposed—in a controlled setting—to forbidden foods or situations where they would ordinarily lose control, vomit, or refuse to eat. The therapist then helps the patient develop appropriate responses to the situation.

Psychoeducation and Group Therapy Psychoeducation is usually delivered in a group setting and consists of educating patients about eating disorders and strategies to treat the disorders. Psychoeducation usually follows principles of cognitive behavioral therapy and may be sufficient for some patients to overcome their disorder without the need for individual counseling. Group therapy differs from psychoeducation in that psychoeducation is used primarily for educating patients and group therapy allows for more discussion and sharing of ideas, where patients can learn from each other. In either case, the group setting helps reduce the patient's feelings of shame, guilt, and isolation.

Psychotherapy focuses on identifying and modifying the interpersonal problems thought to contribute to the eating disorder. Such problems might include underlying grief, disputes with significant others, difficulties forming or maintaining relationships, and difficulty coping with life transitions—such as adolescence and emerging sexuality.

Family Therapy Involving parents, spouses, or other family members in therapy is helpful to increase the patient's support at home and address underlying conflicts. The younger the patient or the more dependent the patient is on family members, the more important it is for family members to be involved.

Pharmacotherapy Since the psychological disturbances of individuals with eating disorders resemble other psychological conditions known to respond to medication, it is reasonable to hypothesize that antipsychotic medications would reduce patients' preoccupation with weight, shape, and food. However, double-blind trials failed to show any benefit of pharmacotherapy specifically for patients with anorexia nervosa. In contrast, antidepressant medications have been shown to improve mood and decrease preoccupation with shape and weight in patients with bulimia nervosa. Although a high proportion of patients with bulimia nervosa have mood disturbances, benefits have been seen in both depressed and non depressed patients with bulimia nervosa (Walsch, 1995).

Pharmacotherapy may be helpful over the short-term for patients with bulimia nervosa, but it is unclear whether benefits can be sustained over several weeks of continued medication and even less clear if any benefits can be maintained over the long-term. Thus, pharmacotherapy for treatment of eating disorders should only be used in conjunction with other approaches and should be dictating by clinical features of the patient and the physician's judgement (Walsch, 1995).

A Stepped-Care Approach As with obesity treatment, conservative treatment for management of eating disorders should be tried first and progress to more intensive and aggressive treatment with more medical risk or inadequate response to conservative treatment. Some individuals in acute medical danger are immediate candidates for hospitalization. For other individuals, psychoeducation or guided self-help may be enough to allow the patient full recovery. For patients who do not respond to education alone, full cognitive behavioral therapy might be the next step, followed by pharmacotherapy or hospitalization for those who fail to respond.

Inpatient Versus Outpatient Therapy

Inpatient care has long been used to treat eating disorders, However, more outpatient or day-hospital facilities are being developed to treat these disorders, and the trend is to provide more treatment in the outpatient setting.

Inpatient treatment is the most intensive approach to treating eating disorders and is most often used in patients with anorexia nervosa. Indications for inpatient treatment include

- Serious physical complications or risk of suicide
- Very low body weight and other medical complications
- Lack of response to outpatient treatment
- Outpatient treatment is not available
- Severe behavioral disturbance
- The need for separation from the family or partner (Fichter,1995)

Serious physical complications include anemia, edema, cachexia, or acute dilation of the stomach and danger of rupture. Often these problems, not the eating disorder itself, are what brings the patient to seek medical attention. Other medical risks include electrolyte disturbances or electrocardiogram changes.

Some individuals fail to respond to outpatient programs or confront a temporary crisis. For others, simply being in a new environment where positive change is reinforced can help patients gain control over their eating. Treatment may also be necessary for some patients who deny their conditions exists.

Whenever possible, inpatient and outpatient treatment should be coordinated to provide the patient as much continuity of care as possible and to provide a smooth transition. In most cases, continued therapy and follow-up is needed over the long term for the patient to make a full recovery.

The next chapter describes components of healthy eating that should be used as an ultimate target for all individuals—including those recovering from obesity or an eating disorder.

EXAM QUESTIONS

CHAPTER 6
Questions 40–46

40. Optimal body weight can be defined as

    a. body weight at age 18

    b. desirable body weight as determined in weight-for-height tables

    c. body mass index of 20 to 23

    d. the most favorable weight for an individual as determined by a variety of factors

41. Which of the following should be a primary consideration in choosing a weight-loss program?

    a. quick weight loss offered

    b. testimonials of other patients

    c. soundness and safety of the program

    d. patient's current calorie intake level

42. What type of weight-loss programs include individual counseling with health care professionals as well as multidisciplinary group programs?

    a. nonclinical programs

    b. clinical programs

    c. do-it-yourself programs

    d. self-directed programs

43. Balanced-deficit diets usually provide what number of calories daily?

    a. less than 500

    b. 500 to 800

    c. 800 to 1,200

    d. 1,200 or more

44. A type of aggressive therapy for obesity treatment is

    a. very low-calorie diet

    b. balanced-deficit diets

    c. behavior modification

    d. exercise

45. Which of the following is true regarding management goals for patients with eating disorders?

    a. Nutrition therapy should be postponed until psychological therapy is completed.

    b. Psychological therapy should be postponed until nutrition therapy is completed.

    c. Psychological therapy should be started immediately, followed by gradual introduction of nutrition therapy as the underlying causes of the eating disorder are addressed.

    d. Nutrition therapy should be started immediately, followed by gradual introduction of psychological therapy as the patients medical and nutrition status begin to stabilize.

46. Cognitive behavioral therapy for patients with eating disorders

    a. is based on the view that cognitions cause faulty food selection, causing the patient to lose weight

    b. is based on the view that certain cognitive characteristics interact with physiological and psychological mechanisms to foster and maintain the eating disorder

    c. consists of educating patients about eating disorders and strategies to treat the disorder

    d. focuses on identifying and modifying the interpersonal problems thought to contribute to the eating disorder

CHAPTER 7

GUIDELINES FOR HEALTHY EATING

CHAPTER OBJECTIVE

After reading this chapter, you will be able to recognize components of a healthy and nutritionally adequate eating plan.

LEARNING OBJECTIVES

After studying this chapter, you will be able to

1. Identify nutritional components of the diet, including carbohydrate, fat, protein, fiber, vitamins, and minerals.

2. Recognize the sound dietary principles for healthy eating.

3. Specify recommended types and amounts of foods that provide the foundation for healthy eating.

4. Specify meanings of descriptive terms used on food labels.

INTRODUCTION

A healthy and nutritionally sound diet is an ultimate goal for all types of treatments for both obesity and eating disorders. Although more aggressive treatment approaches for obesity severely limit food intake and initial therapy for eating disorders may not be completely nutritionally balanced, all weight management approaches should eventually teach patients to select and plan a nutritionally-balanced diet.

COMPONENTS OF GOOD NUTRITION

Good nutrition means providing the body with the right balance of nutrients for optimal functioning. Although the human body has an amazing ability to synthesize hundreds of complex chemicals it needs for proper functioning, some chemicals must be provided as raw materials to make other chemicals.

The chemicals—or nutrients—the body needs for functioning are composed of two main types of nutrients: macronutrients and micronutrients. The macronutrients are proteins, carbohydrates, and fats. Among other functions, these nutrients provide the body with calories that can be burned for fuel. Although not essential, alcohol also provides calories. The micronutrients include vitamins and minerals. Vitamins and minerals do not provide calories but are essential for life, as is water.

Of the macronutrients, fat is the most concentrated source of calories. Fat provides nine calories per gram compared with four calories per gram for carbohydratse and proteins. Alcohol is also a fairly concentrated source of calories providing seven calories per gram.

All three macronutrients—carbohydrates, proteins, and fats—can be metabolized to release energy. In most people's diets, carbohydrates and fats are the primary sources of energy, which allows the body to use protein for synthesis and maintenance of body systems. When carbohydrates and fats are not available for energy from food, the body turns to its own stores of fat, dietary protein, and finally uses its own tissue to meet energy needs.

Proteins

Proteins make up the major structural components of animal cells and are nicknamed "the building blocks of life." Protein is the only substance capable of building and repairing cells and tissues and is the major building material for muscles, blood, skin, nails, and internal organs—including the heart and brain.

Different proteins are formed from different combinations of amino acids strung together like links on a chain and then wound into various shapes. The body is able to convert some amino acids into other amino acids, but there are eight essential amino acids that must be supplied in the diet of humans.

Animal proteins in meat, poultry, fish, eggs, milk, and cheese contain all the essential amino acids and are considered high-quality proteins. Plant proteins do not contain all the essential amino acids but can be combined with other plant proteins eaten throughout the day to provide complete protein.

In general, combining foods in two of the following three plant food groups—dried beans and peas, grain products, or nuts and seeds—will yield complete protein. Examples of such combinations include a peanut butter and jelly sandwich or a beans and rice dish. Combining a small amount of animal protein with a plant protein will also yield complete the plant protein. Examples of this type of combination would be a cheese sandwich or split pea soup with ham.

Recent research indicates that most individuals do not need to eat complementary protein foods at the same time but rather just within the same day to benefit from the amino acids in each. Exceptions might be for very young children, individuals who are extremely undernourished (such as those with severe eating disorders), or individuals with higher nutrient needs, such as pregnant or lactating women.

In a balanced diet, protein should provide 12-20 percent of calories. However, many Americans eat almost twice as much protein as needed. In sedentary individuals, excessive consumption of animal foods that are high in protein but also high in fat (such as fatty cuts of red meat, fried meats, whole milk, and high-fat cheeses) can lead to obesity and other healthy problems (Bray, 1985). High protein intake also decreases calcium absorption, contributing to osteoporosis—a condition in which the bones become brittle and break easily.

Carbohydrates

Contrary to popular belief, carbohydrates are not fattening. Carbohydrates contain less than one-half the calories of fat per equal weight unit. There are two main types of carbohydrates: simple and complex. Simple carbohydrates include naturally occurring sugars found in fruits, vegetables, and milk; and refined sugars like sucrose. Complex carbohydrates include starch and dietary fiber.

Dietary fiber promotes laxation and improves several metabolic functions in the body but is not fully digested and thus provides minimal calories. The two main types of dietary fiber—water soluble and water insoluble—have different benefits to the body. Insoluble fiber is found in whole wheat and most other types of whole cereal grains. Soluble fiber is found in dried beans and peas and oat products. Fruits and vegetables contain both soluble and insoluble fiber.

Insoluble fiber increases stool bulk and aids in regularity. Soluble fiber has been shown to help reduce blood fat levels, help control blood sugar levels, and contribute to a feeling of fullness.

Carbohydrates are the body's preferred fuel source. Starches and sugars are broken down during digestion into small molecules that can be absorbed from the bloodstream and transported to cells. Glucose, a simple carbohydrate, is the main product of these digestive processes. The brain relies almost solely on glucose to provide it with fuel.

Starches from grains and root vegetables have traditionally been man's main source of carbohydrates. Carbohydrates generally make up about 45 to 50 percent of calories in a typical American diet. However, recommended levels of carbohydrate intake are 55 to 60 percent of calories. Therefore, Americans need to eat more carbohydrates__rich foods such as fruits, vegetables, grain products, and dried beans and peas.

Fats

Despite the negative image, some dietary fat is essential to life. Fats are made up of long chains of chemicals called fatty acids, which are chemically bonded to a molecule of glycerol. During digestion, these complex fats are broken down into simpler substances that can be absorbed through the digestive tract, transported to cells, and then used for energy or recombined into fat for storage.

Fats are the most concentrated form of energy available to the body and are an ideal way to store energy. If we had to store all our extra energy in the form of carbohydrates, we wouldn't be able to move. Some stored fat is essential for good health. Stored fat cushions organs, provides a ready energy source during stress, and helps insulate the body from environmental changes. Fat keeps the skin soft and supple, contributes to healthy hair, provides lubrication, and helps the body use the fat-soluble vitamins.

Although some fat is needed in the diet, most Americans eat too much fat. The typical American diet contains 35 to 40 percent or more of calories as fat, whereas the recommended amount is no more than 30 percent of calories as fat. Fortunately, the foods high in complex carbohydrates and naturally occurring sugars that American need to eat more of are also low in fat.

Plant and animal foods both contain fat. There are three main types of fats in the diet—saturated fats, monounsaturated fats, and polyunsaturated fats. Saturated fats are solid at room temperature and contain no double bonds between carbon atoms. Animal fats are generally saturated, with the exception of palm and coconut oil, which are also saturated. Saturated fats are the type most prone to raising blood cholesterol levels and clogging arteries.

Monounsaturated fats contain one double bond between carbon atoms. Monounsaturated fats are liquid at room temperature and may help lower blood cholesterol levels. Olive oil and canola oil are good sources of monounsaturated fats.

Polyunsaturated fats contain multiple double bonds between carbon atoms and are also liquid at room temperature. Most plant oils such as corn, safflower, soybean and sunflower oil are polyunsaturated. However, solid margarines and shortenings made from plant oils have been partially hydrogenated—that is hydrogen atoms have been added back to where the double bonds used to be—making these fats more like saturated fats. Thus liquid or tub margarines are preferable to stick margarines.

Another type of polyunsaturated fats, omega-3 fatty acids, are found in fish oils. The omega-3 fatty acids are one of the few types of unsaturated fats of animal origin. Many studies show that omega-3 fatty acids lower blood triglyceride levels dramatically and blood cholesterol levels modestly. They may also lower risk of heart disease by prolonging clotting time. Fatty fish like salmon, mackerel, haddock, trout and herring are rich in omega-3 fatty acids.

Although monounsaturated fats and polyunsaturated fats do not raise blood cholesterol levels like saturated fats do, they are still fats and are still very concentrated sources of calories. Americans need to reduce total fat as well as saturated fat intake.

Cholesterol is a fat-like substance that is essential for many body functions. It is not really a nutrient since our bodies can make cholesterol also. But when we eat too much cholesterol and saturated fat, our bodies also make even more cholesterol, raising blood cholesterol levels and increasing risk for heart disease.

Cholesterol is found only in animal foods—plant foods contain no cholesterol. Egg yolks and organ meats are particularly concentrated sources of cholesterol. Fattier cuts of red meat and high-fat dairy products are also high in cholesterol. Shellfish such as shrimp, crab, and lobster are not high in cholesterol, as was previously thought.

Alcohol

Alcohol provides seven calories per gram, so it is a fairly concentrated source of calories. Alcoholic beverages provide almost no vitamins or minerals, contain many calories, and are poor choices for individuals trying to lose weight or stabilize eating. Alcoholic beverages often replace other more nutritious foods, leading to poor nutritional content of the diet. In addition, alcohol can raise blood triglyceride levels, which may be a risk factor for heart disease in certain people.

Some studies in the past have suggested that drinking a small amount of alcohol each day raises HDL cholesterol levels, which protect against heart disease. However, recent studies have cast doubt on this theory. The negative effects of alcohol probably outweigh any possible positive effects. Women who are pregnant or trying to conceive should avoid alcohol entirely, since even modest alcohol use during pregnancy can cause birth defects.

Vitamins and Minerals

Vitamins and minerals are needed by the body in small amounts but provide no calories. Vitamins are organic substances needed for special metabolic processes or to prevent deficiencies that cannot be manufactured by the body and must be supplied through food.

Vitamins are usually grouped according to solubility. The fat-soluble vitamins—A, D, E, and K—are closely associated with fats in foods and the body and build up to toxic levels in the body if consumed in excess, including consumption through vitamin supplementation. The water-soluble vitamins—B complex and C—are absorbed, transported, and excreted in the body.

Food sources of vitamins and minerals are shown in *Table 7.1*. Minerals are single inorganic elements essential to life. About 4 percent of the body is composed of minerals. Calcium and phosphorus are essential for healthy bones and teeth. Iron is a key component in hemoglobin. Iodine is a key component in thyroxine. Many enzymes have mineral elements, such as copper, zinc, and molybdenum, or they may require the presence of minerals such as magnesium to complete chemical reactions. Food sources of minerals are also shown in *Table 7.1*.

Actual diseases caused by vitamin or mineral deficiencies are rare in America. Although many Americans take vitamin and mineral supplements, there is no evidence that taking more than the required amount of vitamin or mineral will improve health. Taking too much of certain vitamins or minerals can also be harmful. If use of a vitamin or mineral supplement is indicated, patients should be counseled to select one with a broad base of vitamins and minerals provided at low doses—at approximately 100 percent of the Recommended Dietary Allowances, or RDAs (*Table 7.2*).

The RDAs are defined as "the level of intake of

TABLE 7.1 Food Sources of Vitamins and Minerals

FOODS RICH IN VITAMINS

Vitamin C: Citrus fruits, cantaloupe, strawberries, broccoli, green leafy vegetables, tomatoes

B VITAMINS:

Thiamine (B_1): Dried peas and beans, meats (especially pork), cereals (whole-grain or enriched), nuts

Riboflavin (B_2): Liver, milk, cheese, eggs, green leafy vegetables

Niacin: Liver, meats, dried peas and beans, cereals (whole-grain or enriched)

Pyridoxine (B_6): Liver, meats, wheat germ, whole-grain cereals

Folic acid: Liver, yeast, green leafy vegetables, dried peas and beans, nuts, whole-grain cereals

Cobalamin (B12): Liver and other organ meats, meats, eggs, milk, and milk products

Vitamin A: Liver, butter, eggs, whole milk, green and yellow vegetables

Vitamin D: Fish liver oils, milk fortified with vitamin D, sunlight

Vitamin E: Wheat germ, whole grains, vegetable oils, eggs, whole milk, liver

Vitamin K: Green leafy vegetables, egg yolk, soybean oil, liver

FOODS RICH IN MINERALS

Calcium: Milk, cheese, sardines, ice cream, green leafy vegetables (except for spinach, beet greens, and chard)

Phosphorus: Liver, milk, meat, cheese, cereals, eggs

Iodine: Seafood, vegetables (grown in soil with adequate iodine levels), iodized salt

Iron: Liver, meat, dried fruits, green leafy vegetables

Magnesium: Green leafy vegetables, nuts, whole-grain cereals; dried peas and beans

Potassium: Bananas, oranges, tomatoes, potatoes, broccoli, and some meats

Zinc: Eggs, oysters, liver, meats, poultry, legumes, and nuts

Chromium: Brewer's yeast, grain and cereal products

---

essential nutrients that, on the basis of scientific knowledge, are judged by the Food and Nutrition Board to be adequate to meet the known nutrient needs of practically all healthy persons (Food and Nutrition Board of the National Research Council, 1989).

As shown in *Table 7.2* the RDAs vary according to age groups, with separate categories for pregnant and lactating women. In addition to the RDAs, the Food and Nutrition Board also establishes estimated safe and adequate daily intake of certain vitamins and minerals *(Table 7.3)*. The board makes such estimations when enough data are available to set safe ranges but not absolute requirements. The RDAs can serve as a standard for evaluating the nutritional adequacy of diets.

Water

Water, the most plentiful compound in the body, is often overlooked. The body is composed of 50 to 75 percent water. This remarkable fluid is not only the major ingredient in blood, but is also activity involved in nearly every body function. Water carries and supplies nutrients, participates in chemical reactions, disposes of waste products, regulates the body's temperature. While men and women can exist for weeks without food, most people can't survive longer than 10 days without water.

Each day the body loses large amounts of water through breathing, perspiring, urinating, and other body processes. Thus fluid loss needs to be replaced. Six to eight glasses of fluid daily are recommended, with greater amounts in very hot weather or during strenuous exercise.

TABLE 7.2 Recommended Daily Allowances

Category / Age (years) or Condition	Infants		Children			Males					Females					Pregnant	Lactating	
	0.0–0.5	0.5–1.0	1–3	4–6	7–10	11–14	15–18	19–24	25–50	51+	11–14	15–18	19–24	25–50	51+		1st 6mo.	2nd 6mo.
Weight[b] (kg)	6	9	13	20	28	45	66	72	79	77	46	55	58	63	65			
Weight (lb)	13	20	29	44	62	99	145	160	174	170	101	120	128	138	143			
Height[b] (cm)	60	71	90	112	132	157	176	177	176	173	157	163	164	163	160			
(inches)	24	28	35	44	52	62	69	70	70	68	62	64	65	64	63			
Protein (g)	13	14	16	24	28	45	59	58	63	63	46	44	46	50	50	60	65	62
Fat-Soluble Vitamins																		
Vitamin A (μg RE)[c]	375	375	400	500	700	1,000	1,000	1,000	1,000	1,000	800	800	800	800	800	800	1,300	1,200
Vitamin D (μg)[d]	7.5	10	10	10	10	10	10	10	5	5	10	10	10	5	5	10	10	10
Vitamin E (mg α-TE)[e]	3	4	6	7	7	10	10	10	10	10	8	8	8	8	8	10	12	11
Vitamin K (μg)	5	10	15	20	30	45	65	70	80	80	45	55	60	65	65	65	65	65
Water-Soluble Vitamins																		
Vitamin C (mg)	30	35	40	45	45	50	60	60	60	60	50	60	60	60	60	70	95	90
Thiamin (mg)	0.3	0.4	0.7	0.9	1.0	1.3	1.5	1.5	1.5	1.2	1.1	1.1	1.1	1.1	1.0	1.5	1.6	1.6
Riboflavin (mg)	0.4	0.5	0.8	1.1	1.2	1.5	1.8	1.7	1.7	1.4	1.3	1.3	1.3	1.3	1.2	1.6	1.8	1.7
Niacin (mg NE)[f]	5	6	9	12	13	17	20	19	19	15	15	15	15	15	13	17	20	20
Vitamin B$_6$ (mg)	0.3	0.6	1.0	1.1	1.4	1.7	2.0	2.0	2.0	2.0	1.4	1.5	1.6	1.6	1.6	2.2	2.1	2.1
Folate (μg)	25	35	50	75	100	150	200	200	200	200	150	180	180	180	180	400	280	260
Vitamin B$_{12}$ (μg)	0.3	0.5	0.7	1.0	1.4	2.0	2.0	2.0	2.0	2.0	2.0	2.0	2.0	2.0	2.0	2.2	2.6	2.6
Minerals																		
Calcium (mg)	400	600	800	800	800	1,200	1,200	1,200	800	800	1,200	1,200	1,200	800	800	1,200	1,200	1,200
Phosphorus (mg)	300	500	800	800	800	1,200	1,200	1,200	800	800	1,200	1,200	1,200	800	800	1,200	1,200	1,200
Magnesium (mg)	40	60	80	120	170	270	400	350	350	350	280	300	280	280	280	320	355	340
Iron (mg)	6	10	10	10	10	12	12	10	10	10	15	15	15	15	10	30	15	15
Zinc (mg)	5	5	10	10	10	15	15	15	15	15	12	12	12	12	12	15	19	16
Iodine (μg)	40	50	70	90	120	150	150	150	150	150	150	150	150	150	150	175	200	200
Selenium (μg)	10	15	20	20	30	40	50	70	70	70	45	50	55	55	55	65	75	75

a The allowances, expressed as average daily intake over time, are intended to provide for individual variations among most normal persons as they live in the United States under usual environmental stresses. Diets should be based on a variety of common foods in order to provide other nutrients for which human requirements have been less well defined. See text for detailed discussion of allowances and of nutrients not tabulated.

b Weights and heights of Reference Adults are actual medians for the U.S. population of the designated age, as reported by NHANES II. The median weights and heights of those under 19 years of age were taken from Hamill et al. (1979). The use of those figures does not imply that the height-to-weight ratios are ideal.

c Retinol equivalents. 1 retinol equivalent = 1 μg retinol or 6 μg ß-carotene. See text for calculation of vitamin A activity of diets as retinol equivalents.

d As cholecalciferol. 10 μg cholecalciferol = 400 IU of vitamin D.

e α-Tocopherol equivalents. 1 mg d-α tocopherol = 1 α-TE. See text for variation in allowances and calculation of vitamin E activity of the diet as α-tocopherol equivalents.

f 1 NE (niacin equivalent) is equal to 1 mg of niacin or 60 mg of dietary tryptophan.

Source: Food and Nutrition Board, National Research Council. Reprinted with permission from *Recommended Dietary Allowance, 10th Edition.* Copyright 1989 by the National Academy of Sciences. Courtesy of the National Academy Press, Washington, D.C.

DIETARY GUIDELINES FOR AMERICANS

The U.S. Departments of Agriculture and Health and Human Services (1995) recently updated their guidelines to promote healthy eating for Americans. These seven guidelines are similar to those that were first published in the late 1970s and have been updated regularly as experts learn more about nutrition and disease. The seven current guidelines are

1. **Eat a variety of foods.**

No single type of food supplies all the essential nutrients in the amounts needed. Variety in the diet is so important that it should be repeatedly emphasized. Variety helps maximize the chances that all the essential nutrients will be included in the diet and also minimizes the chances that any one mineral or nutrient will be consumed in excess.

2. **Balance the food you eat with physical activity—maintain or improve your weight.**

Many people gradually gain weight in adulthood, which contributes to chronic conditions such as high blood pressure, heart disease, stroke, type II diabetes, certain cancers, and other illnesses. Calories taken in the diet must be balanced against calories expended in physical activity to adjust the individual's weight as needed. For most individuals needing to lose weight, gradual weight loss through a balanced low-calorie diet and increased physical activity is recommended.

3. **Choose a diet with plenty of grain products, vegetables, and fruits.**

Grains, vegetables, and fruits provide vitamins, minerals, carbohydrates, and dietary fiber. They are also low in fat, saturated fat and cholesterol. These foods should provide the foundation for any healthy diet.

Adults are advised to eat at least three servings of vegetables, two servings of fruits, and six servings daily of grain products such as breads, cereals, pasta and rice. Whenever possible, whole grain products should be chosen to increase fiber intake. Dried beans and peas are also rich in carbohydrate and fiber and low in fat.

4. Choose a diet low in fat, saturated fat, and cholesterol.

Moderate intake of fat and cholesterol is a sensible approach. People don't have to eliminate certain foods from their diet. Rather, they should eat foods high in fat and cholesterol in moderation.

Here are some hints to reduce fat and cholesterol intake

Fats and Oils

- Use fats and oils sparingly in cooking.
- Use small amounts of salad dressings and spreads.
- Choose liquid vegetables oils.

- Read labels.

Meat, poultry, fish, dry beans and eggs

- Eat two to three servings, or about six ounces daily.
- Trim fat from meat and take skin off poultry.
- Use dried beans and peas in place of meat occasionally.
- Use egg yolks and organ meats moderately.

Milk and milk products

- Have two to three servings daily (one serving equals 1 cup of milk or yogurt or 1½ ounce cheese).
- Choose skim, low-fat, or fat-free products.

5. Choose a diet moderate in sugars.

Sugars are a source of carbohydrate. They are added to foods and also occur naturally in foods.

TABLE 7.3
Estimated Safe and Adequate Daily Dietary Intakes of Selected Vitamins and Minerals[a]

VITAMINS

Category	Age (Years)	Biotin (µg)	Panthothenic Acid (mg)
Infants	0–0.5	10	2
	0.5–1	15	3
Children and adolescents	1–3	20	3
	4–6	25	3–4
	7–10	30	4–5
	11+	30–100	4–7
Adults		30–100	4–7

TRACE ELEMENTS[b]

Category	Age (years)	Copper (mg)	Manganese (mg)	Flouride (mg)	Chromium (µg)	Molybdenum (µg)
Infants	0–0.5	0.4–0.6	0.3–0.6	0.1–0.5	10–10	15–30
	0.5–1	0.6–0.7	0.6–1.0	0.2–1.0	20–60	20–40
Children and adolescents	1–3	0.7–1.0	1.0–1.5	0.5–1.5	20–80	25–50
	4–6	1.0–1.5	1.5–2.0	1.0–2.5	30–120	30–75
	7–10	1.0–2.0	2.0–3.0	1.5–2.5	50–200	50–150
	11+	1.5–2.5	2.0–5.0	1.5–2.5	50–200	75–250
Adults		1.5–3.0	2.0–5.0	1.5–4.0	50–200	75–250

a Because there is less information on which to base allowances, these figures are not given in the main table of RDA and are provided here in the form of ranges of recommended intakes.

b Since the toxic levels for many trace elements may be only several times usual intakes, the upper levels for the trace elements given in this table should not be habitually exceeded.

Source: Food and Nutrition Board, National Research Council. Reprinted with permission from *Recommended Dietary Allowances, 10th Edition.* Copyright 1989 by the National Academy of Sciences. Courtesy of the National Academy Press, Washington, D.C.

Examples of sugars added to foods include

- Brown sugar
- Corn sweetener
- Corn syrup
- Fructose
- Fruit juice concentrate
- Glucose (dextrose)
- High-fructose corn syrup
- Honey
- Invert sugar
- Lactose
- Maltose
- Molasses
- Raw sugar
- Sucrose, or table sugar
- Syrup

Although foods high in sugars do not cause hyperactivity or diabetes, they often come packaged with fat in the diet and add extra calories void of nutrients. Most individuals can use modest amounts of sugars in their diet. Individuals on lower-calorie diets will need to use sugars sparingly. Both sugars and starches can promote tooth decay, so proper dental care is important.

To limit sugar in the diet

- Use less of all types of added sugars.
- Select fresh fruits, fruits canned without sugar, or fruits canned in light syrup rather than heavy syrup.
- Read labels for information about sugar added to foods.

6. Choose a diet moderate in salt and sodium.

Both sodium and sodium chloride (table salt) occur naturally in foods and are also added to foods during processing. Most Americans eat too much salt. Excessive sodium intake can contribute to high blood pressure in some people. To consume less salt and sodium

- Read labels to determine the amount of sodium in foods.
- Choose foods lower in sodium, or request less salt in your meals when traveling or eating out.
- If you salt foods in cooking, add small amounts.
- Use spices and herbs instead of salt to flavor foods.
- Choose fresh or frozen plain vegetables instead of canned vegetables.
- When using canned foods, select those low in sodium.
- Choose fresh fruits and vegetables rather than salted snack foods.

7. If you drink alcoholic beverages, do so in moderation

Alcoholic beverages contain calories but are virtually void of nutrients. If adults decide to drink alcoholic beverages, no more than one drink a day is recommended for women and no more than two a day for men. One drink is considered 12 ounces of beer, five ounces of wine, or $1\frac{1}{2}$ ounces of distilled spirits (80 proof).

Some people should not drink alcoholic beverages at all. These include

- Women who are pregnant or trying to conceive
- Individuals who are planning to drive or do another activity that requires concentration
- Individuals taking certain medicines
- Individuals who cannot control their drinking
- Children and adolescents

FIGURE 7.1 The Food Guide Pyramid

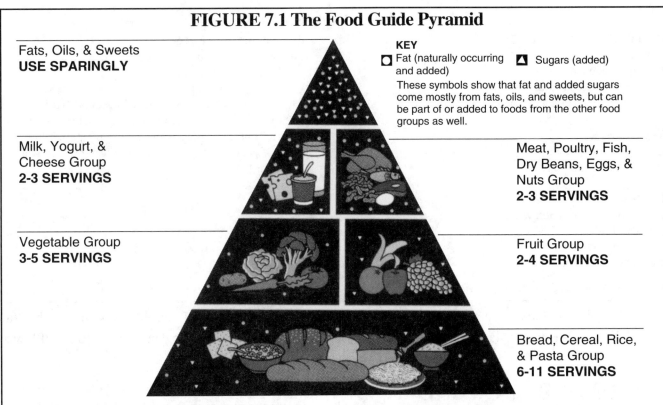

Fats, Oils, & Sweets
USE SPARINGLY

KEY
☐ Fat (naturally occurring and added)   ▲ Sugars (added)

These symbols show that fat and added sugars come mostly from fats, oils, and sweets, but can be part of or added to foods from the other food groups as well.

Milk, Yogurt, & Cheese Group
2-3 SERVINGS

Meat, Poultry, Fish, Dry Beans, Eggs, & Nuts Group
2-3 SERVINGS

Vegetable Group
3-5 SERVINGS

Fruit Group
2-4 SERVINGS

Bread, Cereal, Rice, & Pasta Group
6-11 SERVINGS

Use the Food Guide Pyramid to help you eat better every day ... the Dietary Guidelines way. Start with plenty of breads, cereals, rice, and pasta; vegetables; and fruits. Add two to three servings from the milk group and two to three servings from the meat group.

Each of these food groups provides some, but not all, of the nutrients you need. No one food group is more important than another—for good health you need them all. Go easy on fats, oils, and sweets, the foods in the small tip of the Pyramid.

Source: U.S. Department of Agriculture, Human Nutrition Information Service, August 1992, Leaflet No. 572.

FOUNDATIONS OF HEALTHY EATING: THE FOOD GUIDE PYRAMID

The U.S. Department of Agriculture (1992) introduced a new food guide to replace the basic four food groups and serve as a guide for implementing the Dietary Guidelines for Americans. As shown in *Figure 7.1*, the pyramid recommends ample servings of grains, fruits, and vegetables and more limited servings of dairy products, protein foods, fats.

The Food Guide Pyramid emphasizes that breads, cereals, rice and pastas; fruits; and vegetables are the foundations for health eating and should be consumed in the largest quantities. Ranges are given for intake from each group shown in the Food Guide Pyramid. Individuals with lower calorie needs—such as smaller individuals, some older individuals, and those needing to lose weight—will need to choose the lower number of servings recommended daily (providing about 1,600 calories daily). Individuals with higher calorie needs—such as very active individuals or adolescents—will need to choose the higher number (providing about 2,800 calories daily).

While some patients may be surprised by the quantities of food suggested by this guide, when they eat less fat, they will find that they can eat a much greater volume of food for fewer calories. For controlling calories, choose lower-calorie foods in each group and limit the top group—fats, sweets, and oils. *Table 7.4* shows what counts as a serving for each food group.

TABLE 7.4 What Counts as a Serving?

Breads, Cereal, Rice, and Pasta
1 slice of bread
1/2 cup of cooked rice or pasta
1/2 cup of cooked cereal
1 ounce of ready-to-eat cereal

Vegetables
1/2 cup of chopped raw or cooked vegetables
1 cup of leafy raw vegetables

Fruits
1 piece of fruit or melon wedge
3/4 cup of juice
1/2 cup of canned fruit
1/4 cup of dried fruit

Milk, Yogurt, and Cheese
1 cup of milk or yogurt
1-1/2 to 2 ounces of cheese

Meat, Poultry, Fish, Dry Beans, Eggs, and Nuts
2-1/2 to 3 ounces of cooked lean meat, poultry, or fish
Count 1/2 cup of cooked beans, or 1 egg, or 2 table-spoons of peanut butter as 1 ounce of lean meat (about 1/3 serving)

Source: U.S. Department of Agriculture, Human Nutrition Information Service, August 1992, Leaflet No. 572.

Table 7.5 shows examples of some healthy daily food choices using the Food Guide Pyramid.

UNDERSTANDING FOOD LABELS

Following the National Nutrition Labeling and Education Act of 1990, a major overhaul of the food labeling system took place. New labeling laws now require labels on virtually all foods. Patients should be encouraged to study labels, particularly for information on type of fat, fat content and calorie content.

Consider the sample food label shown in *Figure 7.2*. The amount of calories in a serving and calories from fat are clearly indicated at the top of the "Nutrition Facts." By dividing fat calories by total calories, patients can easily figure the percentage of calories that come from fat in a particular food.

In *Figure 7.2*, 120 fat calories divided by 260 total calories multiplied by 100 means that 46 percent of this food's calories come from fat.

While a reasonable dietary goal is to keep intake of fat to less than 30 percent of daily calories, this does not mean that every food a patient eats must contain less than 30 percent of calories from fat. If a patient eats foods with a higher fat content, they must be balanced with foods of lower fat content.

Before the new labeling regulations, food manufacturers sometimes made questionable health claims on their products or used terms like "light" or "low" loosely. Under the new regulations, only well-substantiated health claims are allowed on packages, and descriptive terms like "free," "low," "lean," "extra lean," "high," "good source," "reduced," "less," "light," and "more" have specific definitions.

With regard to calorie content, "low" means less than 40 calories. "Reduced" means that the product contains 25 percent fewer calories than the regular food. "Light" means that the product contains one-third fewer calories than the regular food.

Table 7.6 defines descriptive terms used on food labels.

SELECTING HEALTHY FOODS

Selecting healthy food involves much more than just knowledge of what is healthy. Food selection is determined by attitudes, time, availability of foods, and many more factors. To

TABLE 7.5 Examples of Daily Food Choices

EXAMPLES OF DAILY FOOD CHOICES

Food Group	No. of Servings	Serving Size	Some Suggested Foods
Vegetables	3-5	1 cup leafy/raw	Leafy greens, lettuce
		1/2 cup other	Corn, peas, green beans, broccoli, carrots, cabbage, celery, tomato, spinach, squash, bok choy, mushrooms, eggplant, collard and mustard greens
		3/4 cup juice	Tomato juice, vegetable juice
Fruits	2-4	1 piece fruit	Orange, apple, applesauce, pear, banana, grapes, grapefruit, tangerine, plum, peach, strawberries and other berries, melons, kiwi, papaya, mango, lychee
		1/2 cup diced fruit	
		3/4 cup fruit juice	Orange juice, apple juice, grapefruit juice, grape juice, prune juice
Breads, cereals, pasta, grains, dry beans, peas, potatoes, and rice	6-11	1 slice	Wheat, rye or enriched breads/rolls, corn and flour tortillas
		1/2 bun, bagel, muffin	English muffin, bagel, muffin, cornbread
		1 oz. dry cereal	Wheat, corn, oat, rice, bran cereal, or mixed grain cereal
		1/2 cup cooked cereal	Oatmeal, cream of wheat, grits
		1/2 cup dry beans or peas	Kidney beans, lentils, split peas, black-eyed peas
		1/2 cup potatoes	Potato, sweet potato
		1/2 cup rice, noodles, barley, or other grains	Pasta, rice, macaroni, barley, tabbouli
		1/2 cup bean curd	Tofu
Skim/low-fat dairy products	2-3	1 cup skim, 1% milk	Low/nonfat yogurt, skim milk, 1% milk, buttermilk
		1.0 oz low-fat, fat-free cheese	Low-fat cheeses
Lean meat, poultry, and fish		≤6 oz/day Step I Diet	Lean and extra lean cuts of meat, fish, and skinless poultry, such as: sirloin, round steak, skinless chicken, haddock, cod
		≤5 oz/day Step II Diet	
Fats and oils	≤6-8*	1 teaspoon soft margarine	Soft or liquid margarine, vegetable oils
		1 tablespoon salad dressing	
		1 oz nuts	Walnuts, peanuts, almonds, pecans
Eggs		≤4 yolks/week-Step I	Used in preparation of baked products
		≤2 yolks/week-Step II	
Sweets and snack foods		In moderation	Cookies, fortune cookies, pudding, bread pudding, rice pudding, angel food cake, frozen yogurt, candy, punch, carbonated beverages
			Low-fat crackers and popcorn, pretzels, fat-free chips, rice cakes

* Includes fats and oils used in food preparation, also salad dressings and nuts.

Source: National Institutes of Health, National Cholesterol Education Program, 1993.

encourage healthy food selection, nurses and dietitians can encourage patients to plan their meals and snacks, read labels, make desirable selections at the grocery store or restaurant, and focus on healthy cooking methods.

Taking the time to preplan meals saves time later by improving efficiency of grocery shopping and cooking. It also yields the added benefit of greater dietary adherence. When meals and snacks are planned ahead, the patient is more likely to make food selections consistent with his or her meal plan and less likely to eat on impulse. When

meals and snacks are preplanned, the patient knows what the next meal is going to be, can start fixing it in a timely manner, and can have the right ingredients on hand. The patient is less likely to grab whatever comes to mind or sight. Preplanning also allows patients to have nutritious, low-calorie snacks available and to keep problem foods out of the house.

Grocery shopping is a critical point of control for individuals trying to control obesity or an eating disorder. A typical grocery store contains thousands of foods. Diet counselors should emphasize that the

FIGURE 7.2 Sample Food Label

Serving sizes are more consistent across product lines.

Nutrition Facts

Serving Size 1/2 cup (114g)
Servings Per Container 4

New title signals the newly required information.

Amount Per Serving

Calories 90   Calories from Fat 30

Calories from fat are shown to help consumers meet dietary guidelines.

% Daily Value*

The list of nutrients covers those most important to the health of today's consumers.

Total Fat 3g	**5%**
Saturated Fat 0g	**0%**
Cholesterol 0mg	**0%**
Sodium 300mg	**13%**
Total Carbohydrate 13g	**4%**
Dietary Fiber 3g	**12%**
Sugars 3g	
Protein 3g	

%Daily Value shows how a food fits into the overall daily diet.

Vitamin A	80%	Vitamin C	60%
Calcium	4%	Iron	4%

* Percent Daily Values are based on a 2.000 calorie diet. Your daily values may be higher or lower depending on your calorie needs:

	Calories	2000	2500
Total Fat	Less than	65g	80g
Sat Fat	Less than	20g	25g
Cholesterol	Less than	300mg	300mg
Sodium	Less than	2400mg	2400mg
Total Carbohydrate		300g	375g
Fiber		25g	30g

Calories per gram:
Fat 9   •   Carbohydrates 4   •   Protein 4

The label tells the number of calories per gram of fat, carbohydrates and protein.

The daily values on the label are based on a daily diet of 2000 and 2500 calories.

Source: FDA Press Kit, Jan 1992.

TABLE 7.6 Descriptive Terms Used on Food Labels

Nutrient	Free	Low	Reduced/Less/Fewer	Other
All	Synonyms for "Free"; "Free of," "No," "Zero," "Without," "Trivial Source of," "Negligible Source of," "Dietary Insignificant Source of"	Synonyms for "Low": "Contains a Small Amount of," "Low Source of," "Low in"	Synonyms for "Reduced/ Less/Fewer": "Reduced in," "Lower," "Low"	
Total calories	Less than 5 calories/reference serving	Less than 40 calories reference serving	Reduced by at least 25%	
Total fat	Less than 0.5 g/reference serving	3 g or less/reference serving Meal and main dish products: 3 g or less per 100 g product and 30% or less calories from fat	Reduced by at least 25%	"___% Fat Free," "___% Lean," must meet requirements for "Low Fat"
Saturated fat	Less than 0.5 g/reference serving, levels of trans fatty acids must be 1% or less of total fat	1 g or less/reference serving and 15% or less of calories from saturated fatty acids Meal and main dish products: 1 g or less per 100 g, and less than 10% of calories from saturated fat	Reduced by at least 25%	
Cholesterol	Less than 2 mg/reference serving; saturated fat content must be 2 g or less	20 mg or less/reference serving; saturated fat content must be 2 g or less per serving Meal and main dish products: 20 mg or less per 100 g, with saturated fat content less than 2 g/100 g	Reduced by at least 25% Contains 2 g or less saturated fat per reference serving	
Sodium	Less than 5 mg/reference serving	140 mg or less/reference serving Meal and main dish products: 140 mg or less/100 g of food	Reduced by at least 25%	"Very Low Sodium," "Very Low in Sodium": 35 mg or less/ reference serving

Source: National Institutes of Health, National Cholesterol Education Program, 1993.

food purchased is the food that will be eaten. If the patient wants to limit or avoid certain foods, they shouldn't be brought into the house. If the patient needs to learn to eat moderate portions of certain foods, then only these portions should be brought into the house at any one time. For patients with eating disorders, preplanning and purchasing only a small amount of a problem food can increase control. If the patient wants to eat more fruits, vegetables and whole-grains, these are the types of foods that should be purchased.

Many fresh fruits and vegetables remain fairly inexpensive all year long. If time is a factor, some precut or presliced healthy foods are worth spending for. Many stores sell prewashed and cut fresh vegetables and boneless, skinless meats.

Several lines of low-calorie frozen dinners are also available. Patients trying to lose weight should be encouraged to select dinners that contain 300 calories or less and 10 grams of fat or less. Patients will also need instruction on rounding out the nutrient content of frozen dinners with fresh fruits, vegetables and nonfat dairy products.

Suggest that the patient preplan meals and shop from a grocery list. Shopping from a list helps reduce impulse buying. Also suggest that the patient avoid shopping when hungry or tired when easiest to lose control.

Since 70 percent of the calorie intake of Americans comes from foods prepared at home, focusing on low-fat cooking methods yields a large payoff for patients trying to limit calories. Some weight loss courses even include cooking demonstrations.

Many Americans are pressed for time and do not want to bother with time-consuming yet healthy recipes. A recent survey noted that 40 percent of Americans don't like the way they eat but think it's too much work to change. Fortunately, many healthy foods require little preparation. Fresh fruits, vegetables, and breads are readily available and easy to prepare.

Here are some tips for healthy food preparation and menu planning

Meat, Poultry and Fish

- Grill, bake, broil or boil instead of fry.
- Trim off all visible fat and remove skin from poultry before cooking.
- Drain meat frequently while cooking.
- Choose leaner cuts of meat.
- Marinade less tender meats in vinegar or wine before.

Dairy Products

- Use skim milk in soups, puddings, and baked products.

- Substitute skimmed milk for evaporated milk in recipes.
- Substitute low-fat cottage cheese or yogurt for sour cream cooking.

Grains

- Use jelly or jam instead of butter on toast.
- Choose hard rolls, bagels, English muffins, or yeast breads in place of sweet rolls, doughnuts, or biscuits.
- Use pasta, rice, or other grains in casseroles and mixed dishes to increase carbohydrate content and decrease fat content.

Vegetables

- Microwave or steam vegetables until just crisp-tender.
- Learn to enjoy the natural flavor of vegetables and avoid drowning them with butter or sauces.
- Eat salads with lemon, vinegar, or nonfat dressings.

Fruit

- Try less common fruits like fresh berries, fresh pineapple, or kiwi fruit for a special treat.
- Use fresh fruit for dessert.

When eating out, nurses should encourage patients to plan ahead. Which restaurant to select is important and patients need to learn to ask questions, make special requests, and emphasize the same types of foods at restaurants as they do at home. Since it is the overall balance of the diet that counts, the more often patients eat out, the more important their selections at restaurants become.

Most restaurants offer at least a few healthy choices on their menus. At fast food restaurants, the plain sandwiches or hamburgers usually contain the least fat and calories. Many fast food restaurants also offer salads, but if you add in the calories in the large packets of dressing, a burger might be a better choice. At a full service restaurant, load up on fresh breads and rolls, pasta and rice dishes, and vegetables. Patients might order a fresh fruit cup to complement their meal. Italian, Mexican, Seafood and Chinese restaurants are but some of the types of restaurants where several lower-calories selections are available.

Patients should also learn to ask questions about how food is prepared and make special requests. Patients can ask that the fish be broiled without added fat, that the butter be left off the vegetables, or that sauces be served on the side.

At a vending machine, patients should be encouraged to choose plain yogurt, a piece of fruit, fruit juice, or crackers.

With microwaves available at many work sites, brown bag lunches can be an extension of home-cooked foods, with soups, stews, casseroles, and salads some of the many choices. The old standby's—sandwiches and fresh fruit and vegeta-bles—are also nutritious low-calorie choices. For variety, try different types of breads and fillings.

When traveling by air, call at least 24 hours ahead of time and ask about heart-healthy or light meals. These often consist of seafood of fruit platters and are often very appealing. When staying in a hotel, bring some food with you. Small boxes of breakfast cereal, instant oatmeal, and fresh fruits travel well.

While all these tips can improve the nutritional value of the diet, it is the balance of food choices over several days that counts. Thus, almost everyone can work in some favorite higher-calorie foods occasionally and still have an overall healthy diet.

The next two chapters describe conservative and aggressive interventions for the management of obesity.

EXAM QUESTIONS

CHAPTER 7
Questions 47–53

47. Which of the following is a macronutrient?

    a. thiamin

    b. iron

    c. protein

    d. vitamin D

48. Which of the following is a micronutrient?

    a. protein

    b. magnesium

    c. carbohydrate

    d. fat

49. Which of the following compounds are considered the building blocks of life?

    a. proteins

    b. carbohydrates

    c. fats

    d. water

50. Which of the following foods contains more water-soluble dietary fiber?

    a. wheat bran

    b. dried beans and peas

    c. rice bran

    d. dried apples

51. How many servings of breads, cereals, rice, and pasta are recommended daily for adults?

    a. 2 to 3

    b. 4

    c. 5

    d. 6 to 11

52. A reasonable dietary goal is to limit the percentage of calories supplied by fat in the diet to

    a. 15 percent

    b. 20 percent

    c. 30 percent

    d. 40 percent

53. The descriptive labeling term "reduced-calorie" means that the food contains what percent fewer calories than the regular food?

    a. 10

    b. 25

    c. 50

    d. 75

CHAPTER 8

INTERVENTION: CONSERVATIVE MANAGEMENT OF OBESITY

CHAPTER OBJECTIVE

After reading this chapter, you will be able to identify types and characteristics of conservative management approaches for obesity.

LEARNING OBJECTIVES

After studying this chapter, you will be able to

1. Differentiate between characteristics of nutritionally sound and unsound diets.

2. Recognize food types and amounts as grouped in the exchange lists.

3. Design meal plans for a balanced calorie-deficit diet based on food exchange lists.

4. Select helpful behavior modification strategies

5. Specify key nutrition counseling strategies for weight control.

INTRODUCTION

Weight management can be broadly grouped into two categories: conservative and aggressive. Within each category there are a variety of types of programs, including self-directed, nonclinical, and clinical.

This chapter will review some characteristics of conservative weight-loss approaches, evaluate some popular weight-loss programs, describe how to calculate a balanced deficit diet using the exchange lists, review some behavior modification techniques, and suggest effective nutrition counseling strategies. Regular physical activity is a critical element in any type of weight-loss approach and is addressed separately in chapter twelve.

WHO IS CONSERVATIVE MANAGEMENT APPROPRIATE FOR?

As reviewed in chapter six, mild to moderate obesity is usually best treated with conservative approaches. Even in moderately obese individuals, conservative approaches should usually be tried before aggressive approaches unless the degree of obesity or significant health risks warrant more aggressive treatment. Mild obesity is defined as a body weight 20 to 39 percent over ideal body weight, or a BMI of 27 to 30. Moderate obesity is defined as a body weight 40 to 100 percent over ideal body weight, or a BMI of 30 to 35. Conservative approaches can also be used as part of a maintenance program for individuals completing more aggressive weight-loss approaches.

THE NURSE'S ROLE

In most instances, a registered dietitian is available to assist with the initial dietary assessment and development of the weight-control plan. As a member of the health care team, however, the nurse will often work with the dietitian to teach and implement this plan. If a registered dietitian is not available, the nurse may be called upon to help develop the weight-loss plan. In either case, nurses must have an understanding of the basic principles in designing a meal plan for weight loss.

CHARACTERISTICS OF BALANCED-DEFICIT DIETS

Balanced-deficit diets are those that provide fewer calories than are usually consumed but not less than 1,200 calories daily. Although most individuals—especially those with health risks—will want to consult their physician before attempting weight loss, balanced-deficit diets are safe for most adults if they provide a variety of foods daily.

In designing and evaluating balanced-deficit diet plans for weight loss, both safety and effectiveness must be considered. Since the ultimate goal of weight-loss approaches is long-term weight maintenance, treatment programs should build on principles of sound nutrition that can be carried into the weight-maintenance phase.

Dwyer (1992) lists four characteristics of balanced-deficit diet plans

1. The diet should provide a safe calorie level.

2. The diet should be nutritionally balanced, with carbohydrates, proteins and fats, provided in the right balance.

3. The overall weight-loss plan should include other components essential to weight control, such as instruction in exercise and behavior modification.

4. The cost of the diet plan should be reasonable.

EVALUATING POPULAR WEIGHT-LOSS PROGRAMS

The two main considerations in evaluating commercial and popular diets are effectiveness and safety. Most commercial weight-loss programs are conservative in nature. However, 50 percent of those entering commercial weight-loss programs drop out within the first six weeks. At 12 weeks, drop-out rate is almost 70 percent (Perri, 1992). Of those who remain in commercial programs for longer periods, weight loss is still often modest and frequently not maintained. The effectiveness of popular diets is usually difficult to evaluate because of their short-lived nature.

Nurses should counsel patients to avoid commercial and popular diets that do not include professional supervision, adjunct exercise or behavior modification, or a maintenance phase. Fad diets that severely restrict intake of certain foods or nutrients should also be avoided. Diets that restrict carbohydrates, salt, or fluids cause rapid weight loss the first few weeks, but the loss is mostly from fluid and will be quickly regained when the patient resumes normal eating.

Dwyer (1992) reviewed popular diets and grouped them into three categories—reasonable, questionable, and unreasonable—according to safety of the calorie level, nutrient composition of the diet, completeness of components of the program other than diet, and cost. The results of Dwyer's review are listed in *Table 8.1.*

TABLE 8.1
Some Reasonable, Questionable, and Unreasonable Diets for the Treatment of Obesity

1200 calories per day or more *Reasonable diets*
I Don't Eat (But I Can't Lose) Weight Control Program
Harvard Square Diet
Red Book Wise Women's Diet
Doctor's Calorie Plus
Behavior Control Diet
California Nutrition Book
California Diet
LEARN Program for Weight Control
Complete University Medical Diet

Questionable diets
Oat and Wheat Bran Health Plan
New Canadian Fiber Diet (DePrey)
Women's Advantage Diet (Mallek)
The 35 Plus Diet for Women
Bad Back Diet Book (Green and Ceresa)
"T" Factor Diet
The Mediterranean Diet
Atkin's Diet Revolution
Nutrition Breakthrough
Dr. Abravanel's Body Type Diet
Doctor's Quick Weight Loss
Pritikin Program Diet
Craig Claibourne's Gourmet Diet
Rechtschaffen Diet
Orthocarbohydrate Diet
Easy No Risk Dict
Slender Now
Never Say Diet
F Plan Diet
Carbohydrate Craver's Diet
Dr. Atkin's Health Revolution
Immune Power
What Your Doctor Didn't Learn in Medical School

800 to 1199 calories per day *Reasonable diets*
Lean and Green Diet
Hilton Head Metabolism Diet
Weight Watcher's Quick Start Program
Diet Workshop Lo Carbo and Beacon Hill Diets

Questionable diets
Two Day Diet
Rotation Diet
Diet Workshop Wild Weekend
The Hilton Head Over 35 Diet
L. A. Diet
Doctor's Metabolic Diet
No Choice Diet
Woman Doctor's Diet
Southhampton Diet
Bloomingdale Diet
Herbalife Slim Trim Diet
Fit for Life
Thin So Fast (Fades)
The Rice Diet
Beverly Hills Diet

800 calories or less *Reasonable diets (only if administered under medical supervision)*
HMR (Health Management Resources)
Optifast
United Weight Control
New Directions (Ross Laboratories)
Nutrisystem

Questionable diets
Herbalife
Last Chance Diet
Fasting Is A Way of Life

Source: Dwyer, J. T. (1992). "Treatment of obesity: Conventional programs and fad diets." In P. Bjorntorp and B. N. Brodoff (Eds.), *Obesity* (pp.662-676). Philadelphia: J. B. Lippinoott Co. Reprinted with permission.

CALORIE AND NUTRIENT COMPOSITION OF BALANCED-DEFICIT DIETS

One of the first steps in weight reduction in designing a balanced-deficit diet is to establish the number of calories that will lead to a slow but sure rate of weight loss. Although most patients and health care providers wish weight could be lost quicker, a rate of weight loss of one to two pounds weekly is a safe and reasonable goal (American Dietetic Association, 1989).

Most individuals will lose weight faster the first week or two of dieting because of fluid losses.

The difference between the calories expended and the calories ingested is called the calorie deficit. A calorie deficit of 3,500 calories will lead to a loss of one pound of body fat. A patient can expect to lose about one pound per week with a calorie deficit of 500 calories daily ($7 \times 500 = 3{,}500$ calories). A patient can expect to lose about two pounds per week with a calorie deficit of 1,000 calories daily ($7 \times 1{,}000 = 7{,}000$ calories divided by 3,500 calories in a pound = 2 pounds). Since it is very difficult to exercise away 500 or more calories daily, the calorie deficit should ideally be obtained by a combination of cutting calories out of the diet and by increasing physical activity.

One way to determine a calorie level for weight loss is to use the initial dietary assessment. Current calorie intake can be estimated using food records or 24-hour food recalls for typical days. To lose weight, the patient must eat 500 to 1,000 calories less than they currently eat daily, or achieve an equivalent calorie deficit by combining calorie reduction with increased physical activity.

Another approach is to estimate calories to maintain weight using the following figures for varying activity levels

- **Sedentary:** 10–12 calories per pound actual body weight

- **Active:** 13–15 calories per pound actual body weight

- **Very active:** 16–20 calories per pound of actual body weight

Then subtract out 500 to 1,000 calories daily for weight loss.

Most inactive women maintain weight on around 1,800 to 2,000 calories daily. Most inactive men maintain weight on around 2,400 to 2,600 calories daily. (Men usually require more calories than women because they have more lean body mass, which burns more calories.) Therefore most women will lose about a pound a week on 1,200 calories daily, while most men will lose about a pound a week on 1,800 calories daily. If the individual also increases activity, weight losses will be greater.

Determining a calorie level for weight loss is always an estimate. Calorie levels may need adjusting on follow-up visits and as the individual loses weight. Also, different patients differ in their ability to lose weight on a set calorie level because of differences in adherence, physical activity, body metabolism, diet composition, and water balance. Some individuals may also underestimate portion sizes or overestimate physical activity.

Deficit diets should also provide the right balance of carbohydrates, proteins, and fats. Nutritional recommendations for the general population are that carbohydrates should provide about 55 to 60 percent of total calories, fats should provide less than 30 percent of calories, and proteins should make up the difference.

Fat is the most concentrated source of calories, so reducing fat in the diet will help dieters get a greater volume of food for fewer calories. Gram for gram, carbohydrates provide less than one-half the calories of fat, so foods rich in carbohydrates and fiber should be emphasized in a weight-loss program.

Guidelines for appropriate nutrient composition of low-calorie diets are (Dwyer, 1992)

- 100 grams or more of carbohydrates, to spare body protein

- A minimum of about 44 grams of high-quality protein for women and about 56 grams for men

- Less than 30 percent of calories as fat

- 20–30 grams of dietary fiber daily

- Less than 200 milligrams of cholesterol daily

- At least 1 liter of water daily, or 1 ml/calorie/day

- an intake of vitamins and minerals at least equal to values specified by the Recommended Dietary Allowances (see chapter seven).

As the calorie level of the diet decreases, the percentage of calories provided by protein will increase to achieve the minimum recommended level of protein daily. At calorie intakes of less than 1,200, it may be necessary to take a low-dose multivitamin and mineral preparation to achieve adequate intakes of vitamins and minerals.

THE EXCHANGE LISTS FOR WEIGHT MANAGEMENT

To lose weight, some individuals may prefer to count their calorie intake daily and follow the basic recommended number of servings from the food guide pyramid presented in chapter seven. While this approach is also acceptable and teaches principles of sound nutrition for weight maintenance, some individuals do not want to keep track of calories. Some patients also require a more structured diet.

Dietitians and other health care professionals have traditionally used exchange lists in designing individual meal plans for patients. The food exchange lists group foods with similar calorie and nutrient levels together, so one food can be substituted for another in each list. For example, a slice of bread and 1/2 cup of pasta are both on the starch list. Each contain about 80 calories and similar amounts of carbohydrates, vitamins, proteins, and other essential nutrients.

The American Diabetes and Dietetic Associations recently released an updated version of the Food Exchange Lists for Weight Management (1995). A simplified, pictorial versions of these exchange lists called *Eating Healthy Foods* is also available and is especially useful for patients with limited reading skills (The American Diabetes Association and The American Dietetic Association, 1988).

The exchange lists have traditionally divided foods into six main groups: starch, fruit, vegetable, milk, meat, and fat. A seventh group, "other carbohydrates," was added in the latest revision of the exchange lists. This "other carbohydrate" group includes foods like cakes, cookies, doughnuts, fruit juice bars, puddings, and other prepared foods. Foods in this group can be substituted for a starch, fruit, or milk choice, but foods in this group may not contain as many vitamins and minerals as foods in the other groups. They may also count as one or more fat exchanges.

Nurses or dietitians can specify the number of servings a patient should have from each exchange group daily. The approximate calorie and nutrient composition of the diet will be known without the patient having to keep track of calories.

The size of a portion is important, and each serving is one exchange. If the portion is doubled, it equals two exchanges. For example, two slices of whole wheat bread equal two bread exchanges.

The foods in each of the seven exchange lists are shown in *Table 8.2. Table 8.3* gives the calorie and nutrient content of each of the seven exchange groups.

STEPS IN CALCULATING A MEAL PLAN

Calculating meal plans based on the exchange lists can be simplified by following the steps listed below

1. Estimate energy needs for maintenance and subtract 500 to 1,000 calories, but do not go below 1,200 calories without proper medical supervision.

2. Distribute calories into desired percentage of proteins, carbohydrates, and fats. For example, for a diet that supplies 20 percent of calories as protein, 55 percent as carbohydrate, and 25 percent as fat, multiple calorie level by 0.20 for protein, 0.55 for carbohydrate, and 0.25 for fat.

3. Convert calories from proteins, carbohydrates, and fats into grams by dividing protein calories by 4 calories per gram, carbohydrate calories

TABLE 8.2 Exchange Lists Summary Sheet

STARCH LIST

Cereals, grains, pasta, breads, crackers, snacks, starchy vegetables, and cooked dried beans, peas, and lentils are starches. In general, one starch is:

- 1/2 cup of cereal, grain, pasta, or starchy vegetable,
- 1 ounce of a bread product, such as 1 slice of bread,
- 3/4 to 1 ounce of most snack foods. (Some snack foods may also have added fat.)

Nutrition Tips

1. Most starch choices are good sources of B vitamins.
2. Foods made from whole grains are good sources of fiber.
3. Dried beans and peas are a good source of protein and fiber.

Selection Tips

1. Choose starches made with little fat as often as you can.
2. Starchy vegetables prepared with fat count as one starch and one fat.
3. Bagels or muffins can be 2, 3, or 4 ounces in size, and can, therefore, count as 2, 3, or 4 starch choices. Check the size you eat.
4. Dried beans, peas, and lentils are also found on the Meat and Meat Substitutes list.
5. Regular potato chips and tortilla chips are found on the Other Carbohydrates list.
6. Most of the serving sizes are measured after cooking.
7. Always check Nutrition Facts on the food label.

One starch exchange equals 15 grams carbohydrate, 3 grams protein, 0–1 grams fat, and 80 calories.

Bread

Bagel	1/2 (1 oz)
Bread, reduced-calorie	slices (1½ oz)
Bread, white, whole-wheat, pumpernickel, rye	1 slice (1 oz)
Bread sticks, crisp, 4 in. long x 1/2 in	2 (2/3 oz)
English muffin	1/2
Hot dog or hamburger bun	1/2 (1 oz)
Pita, 6 in. across	1/2
Roll, plain, small	1 (1 oz)
Raisin bread, unfrosted	1 slice (1 oz)
Tortilla, corn, 6 in. across	1
Tortilla, flour, 7-8 in. across	1
Waffle, 4 1/2 in. square, reduced-fat	1

Cereals and Grains

Bran cereals	1/2 cup
Bulgur	1/2 cup
Cereals	1/2 cup
Cereals, unsweetened, ready-to-eat	3/4 cup
Cornmeal (dry)	3 Tbsp
Couscous	1/3 cup

Flour (dry)	3 Tbsp
Granola, low-fat	1/4 cup
Grape-Nuts	1/4 cup
Grits	1/2 cup
Kasha	1/2 cup
Millet	1/4 cup
Muesli	1/4 cup
Oats	1/2 cup
Pasta	1/2 cup
Puffed cereal	1½ cups
Rice milk	1/2 cup
Rice, white or brown	1/3 cup
Shredded Wheat	1/2 cup
Sugar-frosted cereal	1/2 cup
Wheat germ	3 Tbsp

Starchy Vegetables

Baked beans	1/3 cup
Corn	1/2 cup
Corn on cob, medium	1 (5 oz)
Mixed vegetables with corn, peas, or pasta	1 cup
Peas, green	1/2 cup
Plantain	1/2 cup
Potato, baked or boiled	1 small (3 oz)
Potato, mashed	1/2 cup
Squash, winter (acorn, butternut)	1 cup
Yam, sweet potato, plain	1/2 cup

Crackers And Snacks

Animal crackers	8
Graham crackers, 2 1/2 in. square	3
Matzoh	3/4 oz
Melba toast	4 slices
Oyster crackers	24
Popcorn (popped, no fat added or low-fat microwave)	3 cups
Pretzels	3/4 oz
Rice cakes, 4 in. across	2
Saltine-type crackers	6
Snack chips, fat-free (tortilla, potato)	15–20 (3/4 oz)
Whole-wheat crackers, no fat added	2–5 (3/4 oz)

Dried Beans, Peas, And Lentils

(Count as 1 starch exchange, plus 1 very lean meat exchange.)

Beans and peas (garbanzo, pinto, kidney, white, split, black-eyed)	1/2 cup
Lima beans	2/3 cup
Lentils	1/2 cup
Miso*	3 Tbsp

Starchy Foods Prepared With Fat

(Count as 1 starch exchange, plus 1 fat exchange.)

Biscuit, 2 1/2 in. across	1
Chow mein noodles	1/2 cup
Corn bread, 2 in. cube	1 (2 oz)
Crackers, round butter type	6
Croutons	1 cup

* = 400 mg or more of sodium per serving.

TABLE 8.2 Exchange Lists Summary Sheet *(Cont.)*

Starchy Foods Prepared With Fat Continued

French-fried potatoes . . . . .16–25 (3 oz)
Granola . . . . .1/4 cup
Muffin, small . . . . .1(1½ oz)
Pancake, 4 in. across 2
Popcorn, microwave . . . . .3 cups
Sandwich crackers, cheese or peanut butter filling 3
Stuffing, bread (prepared) .1/3 cup
Taco shell, 6 in. across 2
Waffle, 4 ½ in. square 1
Whole-wheat crackers, fat added . . . . .4–6 (1 oz)

Some food you buy uncooked will weigh less after you cook it. Starches often swell in cooking, so a small amount of uncooked starch will become a much larger amount of cooked food. The following table shows some of the changes.

Food (Starch Group)	Uncooked	Cooked
Oatmeal	3 Thsp	1/2 cup
Cream of Wheat	2 Tbsp	1/2 cup
Grits	3 Tbsp	1/2 cup
Rice	2 Tbsp	1/3 cup
Spaghetti	1/4 cup	1/2 cup
Noodles	1/3 cup	1/2 cup
Macaroni	1/4 cup	1/2 cup
Dried beans	1/4 cup	1/2 cup
Dried peas	1/4 cup	1/2 cup
Lentils	3 Tbsp	1/2 cup

Common Measurements

3 tsp = 1 Tbsp   4 ounces = 1/2 cup
4 Tbsp = 1/4 cup   8 ounces = 1 cup
5⅓ Tbsp = 1/3 cup . . . . .1 cup = 1/2 pint

FRUIT LIST

Fresh, frozen, canned, and dried fruits and fruit juices are on this list. In general, one fruit exchange is:

- 1 small to medium fresh fruit,
- 1/2 cup of canned or fresh fruit or fruit juice,
- 1/4 cup of dried fruit.

Nutrition Tips

1. Fresh, frozen, and dried fruits have about 2 grains of fiber per choice. Fruit juices contain very little fiber.
2. Citrus fruits, berries, and melons are good sources of vitamin C.

Selection Tips

1. Count 1/2 cup cranberries or rhubarb sweetened with sugar substitutes as free foods.
2. Read the Nutrition Facts on the food label. If one serving has more than 15 grams of carbohydrate, you will need to adjust the size of the serving you eat or drink.
3. Portion sizes for canned fruits are for the fruit and a small amount of juice.
4. Whole fruit is more filling than fruit juice and may be a better choice.
5. Food labels for fruits may contain the words "no sugar added" or "unsweetened." This means that no sucrose

(table sugar) has been added.

6. Generally, fruit canned in extra light syrup has the same amount of carbohydrate per serving as the "no sugar added" or the juice pack. All canned fruits on the fruit list are based on one of these three types of pack.

One fruit exchange equals 15 grams carbohydrate and 60 calories. The weight includes skin, core, seeds, and rind.

Fruit

Apple, unpeeled, small . . . . .1 (4 oz)
Applesauce, unsweetened . . . . .1/2 cup
Apples, dried . . . . .4 rings
Apricots, fresh . . . . .4 whole (5½ oz)
Apricots, dried . . . . .8 halves
Apricots, canned . . . . .1/2 cup
Banana, small . . . . .1(4 oz)
Blackberries . . . . .3/4 cup
Blueberries . . . . .3/4 cup
Cantaloupe, small . . . . . . .1/3 melon (11 oz) or 1 cup cubes
Cherries, sweet, fresh . . . . .12 (3 oz)
Cherries, sweet, canned . . . . .1/2 cup
Dates 3
Figs, fresh . . . . .1½ large or 2 medium (3½ oz)
Figs, dried 1½
Fruit cocktail . . . . .1/2 cup
Grapefruit, large . . . . .1/2 (11 oz)
Grapefruit sections, canned . . . . .3/4 cup
Grapes, small . . . . .17 (3 oz)
Honeydew melon . . . . .1 slice (10 oz) or 1 cup cubes
Kiwi . . . . .1 (3½ oz)
Mandarin oranges, canned . . . . .3/4 cup
Mango, small . . . . .1/2 fruit (5½ oz) or 1/2 cup
Nectarine, small . . . . .1 (5 oz)
Orange, small . . . . .1 (6½ oz)
Papaya . . . . .1/2 fruit (8 oz) or 1 cup cubes
Peach, medium, fresh . . . . .1 (6 oz)
Peaches, canned . . . . .1/2 cup
Pear, large, fresh . . . . .1/2 (4 oz)
Pears, canned . . . . .1/2 cup
Pineapple, fresh . . . . .3/4 cup
Pineapple, canned . . . . .1/2 cup
Plums, small . . . . .2 (5 oz)
Plums, canned . . . . .1/2 cup
Prunes, dried 3
Raisins . . . . .2 Tbsp
Raspberries . . . . .1 cup
Strawberries . . . . .1¼ cup whole berries
Tangerines, small . . . . .2 (8 oz)
Watermelon . . . . .1 slice (13½ oz) or 1¼ cup cubes

Fruit Juice

Apple juice/cider . . . . .1/2 cup
Cranberry juice cocktail . . . . .1/3 cup
Cranberry juice cocktail, reduced-calorie . . . . 1 cup
Fruit juice blends, 100% juice . . . . .1/3 cup
Grape juice . . . . .1/3 cup
Grapefruit juice . . . . .1/2 cup
Orange juice . . . . .1/2 cup
Fruit Juice Continued

TABLE 8.2 Exchange Lists Summary Sheet *(Cont.)*

Pineapple juice . . . . .1/2 cup
Prune juice . . . . .1/3 cup

MILK LIST

Different types of milk and milk products are on this list. Cheeses are on the Meat list and cream and other dairy fats are on the Fat list. Based on the amount of fat they contain, milks are divided into skim/very low-fat milk, low-fat milk, and whole milk. One choice of these includes:

	Carbohydrate (grams)	Protein (grams)	Fat (grams)	Calories
Skim/very low-fat	12	8	0–3	90
Low-fat	12	8	5	120
Whole	12	8	8	150

Nutrition Tips

1. Milk and yogurt are good sources of calcium and protein. Check the food label.
2. The higher the fat content of milk and yogurt, the greater the amount of saturated fat and cholesterol. Choose lower-fat varieties.
3. For those who are lactose intolerant, look for lactose-reduced or lactose-free varieties of milk.

Selection Tips

1. One cup equals 8 fluid ounces or 1/2 pint.
2. Look for chocolate milk, frozen yogurt, and ice cream on the Other Carbohydrates list.
3. Nondairy creamers are on the Free Foods list.
4. Look for rice milk on the Starch list.
5. Look for soy milk on the Medium-fat Meat list.

One milk exchange equals 12 grams carbohydrate and 8 grams protein.

Skim And Very Low-fat Milk

(0-3 grams fat per serving)
Skim milk . . . . .1 cup
1/2% milk . . . . .1 cup
1% milk . . . . .1 cup
Nonfat or low-fat buttermilk .1 cup
Evaporated skim milk . . . . .1/2 cup
Nonfat dry milk . . . . .1/3 cup dry
Plain nonfat yogurt . . . . .3/4 cup
Nonfat or low-fat fruit-flavored yogurt sweetened
with aspartame or with a nonnutritive sweetener . . . . .1 cup

Low-fat

(5 grams fat per serving)
2% milk . . . . .1 cup
Plain low-fat yogurt . . . . .3/4 cup
Sweet acidophilus milk . . . . .1 cup

Whole Milk

(8 grams fat per serving)
Whole milk . . . . 1 cup
Evaporated whole milk . . . . .1/2 cup
Goat's milk . . . . 1 cup
Kefir . . . . 1 cup

OTHER CARBOHYDRATES LIST

You can substitute food choices from this list for a starch, fruit, or milk choice on your meal plan. Some choices will also count as one or more fat choices.

Nutrition Tips

1. These foods can be substituted in your meal plan, even though they contain added sugars or fat. However, they do not contain as many important vitamins and minerals as the choices on the Starch, Fruit, or Milk list.
2. When planning to include these foods in your meal, be sure to include foods from all the lists to eat a balanced meal.

Selection Tips

1. Because many of these foods are concentrated sources of carbohydrate and fat, the portion sizes are often very small.
2. Always check Nutrition Facts on the food label. It will be your most accurate source of information.
3. Many fat-free or reduced-fat products made with fat replacers contain carbohydrate. When eaten in large amounts, they may need to be counted. Talk with your dietitian to determine how to count these in your meal plan.
4. Look for fat-free salad dressings in smaller amounts on the Free Foods list.

One exchange equals 15 grams carbohydrate, or 1 starch, or 1 fruit, or 1 milk.

TABLE 8.2 Exchange Lists Summary Sheet *(Cont.)*

Food	Serving Size	Exchanges Per Serving
Angel food cake, unfrosted	1/12th cake	2 carbohydrates
Brownie, small, unfrosted	2 in. square	1 carbohydrate, 1 fat
Cake, unfrosted	2 in. square	1 carbohydrate, 1 fat
Cake, frosted	2 in. square	2 carbohydrates, 1 fat
Cookie, fat-free	2 small	1 carbohydrate
Cookie or sandwich cookie with creme filling	2 small	1 carbohydrate, 1 fat
Cupcake, frosted	1 small	2 carbohydrates, 1 fat
Cranberry sauce, jellied	1/4 cup	2 carbohydrates
Doughnut, plain cake	1 medium (1½ oz)	1½ carbohydrates, 2 fats
Doughnut, glazed	3¾ in. across (2 oz)	2 carbohydrates, 2 fats
Fruit juice bars, frozen, 100% juice	1 bar (3 oz)	1 carbohydrate
Fruit snacks, chewy (pureed fruit concentrate)	1 roll (3/4 oz)	1 carbohydrate
Fruit spreads, 100% fruit	1 Tbsp	1 carbohydrate
Gelatin, regular	1/2 cup	1 carbohydrate
Gingersnaps	3	1 carbohydrate
Granola bar	1 bar	1 carbohydrate, 1 fat
Granola bar, fat-free	1 bar	2 carbohydrates
Hummus	1/3 cup	1 carbohydrate, 1 fat
Ice cream	1/2 cup	1 carbohydrate, 2 fats
Ice cream, light	1/2 cup	1 carbohydrate, 1 fat
Ice cream, fat-free, no sugar added	1/2 cup	1 carbohydrate
Jam or jelly, regular	1 Tbsp	1 carbohydrate
Milk, chocolate, whole	1 cup	2 carbohydrates, 1 fat
Pie, fruit, 2 crusts	1/6 pie	3 carbohydrate, 2 fats
Pie, pumpkin or custard	1/8 pie	1 carbohydrate, 2 fats
Potato chips	12–18 (1 oz)	1 carbohydrate, 2 fats
Pudding, regular (made with low-fat milk)	1/2 cup	2 carbohydrates
Pudding, sugar-free (made with low-fat milk)	1/2 cup	1 carbohydrate
Salad dressing, fat-free*	1/4 cup	1 carbohydrate
Sherbet, sorbet	1/2 cup	2 carbohydrates
Spaghetti or pasta sauce, canned*	1/2 cup	1 carbohydrate, 1 fat
Sweet roll or Danish	1 (2½ oz)	2½ carbohydrates, 2 fats
Syrup, light	2 Tbsp	1 carbohydrate
Syrup, regular	1 Tbsp	1 carbohydrate
Syrup, regular	1/4 cup	4 carbohydrates
Tortilla chips	6–12 (1 oz)	1 carbohydrate, 2 fats
Yogurt, frozen, low-fat, fat-free	1/3 cup	1 carbohydrate, 0–1 fat
Yogurt, frozen, fat-free, no sugar added	1/2 cup	1 carbohydrate
Yogurt, low-fat with fruit	1 cup	3 carbohydrates, 0–1 fat
Vanilla wafers	5	1 carbohydrate, 1 fat

* = 400 mg or more of sodium per serving.

TABLE 8.2 Exchange Lists Summary Sheet *(Cont.)*

VEGETABLE LIST

Vegetables that contain small amounts of carbohydrates and calories are on this list. Vegetables contain important nutrients. Try to eat at least 2 or 3 vegetable choices each day. In general, one vegetable exchange is:

- 1/2 cup of cooked vegetables or vegetable juice,
- 1 cup of raw vegetables.

If you eat 1 to 2 vegetable choices at a meal or snack, you do not have to count the calories or carbohydrates because they contain small amounts of these nutrients.

Nutrition Tips

1. Fresh and frozen vegetables have less added salt than canned vegetables. Drain and rinse canned vegetables if you want to remove some salt.
2. Choose more dark green and dark yellow vegetables, such as spinach, broccoli, romaine, carrots, chilies, and peppers.
3. Broccoli, brussels sprouts, cauliflower, greens, peppers, spinach, and tomatoes are good sources of vitamin C.
4. Vegetables contain 1 to 4 grams of fiber per serving.

Selection Tips

1. A 1-cup portion of broccoli is a portion about the size of a light bulb.
2. Tomato sauce is different from spaghetti sauce, which is on the Other Carbohydrates list.
3. Canned vegetables and juices are available without added salt.
4. If you eat more than 4 cups of raw vegetables or 2 cups of cooked vegetables at one meal, count them as 1 carbohydrate choice.
5. Starchy vegetables such as corn, peas, winter squash, and potatoes that contain larger amounts of calories and carbohydrates are on the Starch list.

One vegetable exchange equals 5 grams carbohydrate, 2 grams protein, 0 grams fat, and 25 calories.

Artichoke

Artichoke hearts

Asparagus

Beans (green, wax, Italian)

Bean sprouts

Beets

Broccoli

Brussels sprouts

Cabbage

Carrots

Cauliflower

Celery

Cucumber

Eggplant

Green onions or scallions

Greens (collard, kale, mustard, turnip)

Kohlrabi

Leeks

Mixed vegetables (without corn, peas, or pasta)

Mushrooms

Okra

Onions

Pea pods

Peppers (all varieties)

Radishes

Salad greens (endive, escarole, lettuce, romaine, spinach)

Sauerkraut*

Spinach

Summer squash

Tomato

Tomatoes, canned

Tomato sauce*

Tomato/vegetable juice*

Turnips

Water chestnuts

Watercress

Zucchini

MEAT AND MEAT SUBSTITUTES LIST

Meat and meat substitutes that contain both protein and fat are on this list. In general, one meat exchange is:

- 1 oz meat, fish, poultry, or cheese,
- 1/2 cup dried beans.

Based on the amount of fat they contain, meats are divided into very lean, lean, medium-fat, and high-fat lists. This is done so you can see which ones contain the least amount of fat. One ounce (one exchange) of each of these includes:

	Carbohydrate (grams)	Protein (grams)	Fat (grams)	Calories
Very lean	0	7	0–1	35
Lean	0	7	3	55
Medium-fat	0	7	5	75
High-fat	0	7	8	100

Nutrition Tips

1. Choose very lean and lean meat choices whenever possible. Items from the high-fat group are high in saturated fat, cholesterol, and calories and can raise blood cholesterol levels.
2. Meats do not have any fiber.
3. Dried beans, peas, and lentils are good sources of fiber.

* = 400 mg or more of sodium per serving.

TABLE 8.2 Exchange Lists Summary Sheet *(Cont.)*

Nutrition Tips Continued

4. Some processed meats, seafood, and soy products may contain carbohydrate when consumed in large amounts. Check the Nutrition Facts on the label to see if the amount is close to 15 grams. If so, count it as a carbohydrate choice as well as a meat choice.

Selection Tips

1. Weigh meat after cooking and removing bones and fat. Four ounces of raw meat is equal to 3 ounces of cooked meat. Some examples of meat portions are:
    *   1 ounce cheese = 1 meat choice and is about the size of a 1-inch cube
    *   2 ounces meat = 2 meat choices, such as
        1 small chicken leg or thigh
        1/2 cup cottage cheese or tuna
    *   3 ounces meat = 3 meat choices and is about the size of a deck of cards, such as
        1 medium pork chop
        1 small hamburger
        1/2 of a whole chicken breast
        1 unbreaded fish fillet
2. Limit your choices from the high-fat group to three times per week or less.
3. Most grocery stores stock Select and Choice grades of meat. Select grades of meat are the leanest meats. Choice grades contain a moderate amount of fat, and Prime cuts of meat have the highest amount of fat. Restaurants usually serve Prime cuts of meat.
4. "Hamburger" may contain added seasoning and fat, but ground beef does not.
5. Read labels to find products that are low in fat and cholesterol (5 grams or less of fat per serving).
6. Dried beans, peas, and lentils are also found on the Starch list.
7. Peanut butter, in smaller amounts, is also found on the Fats list.
8. Bacon, in smaller amounts, is also found on the Fats list.

Meat Planning Tips

1. Bake, roast, broil, grill, poach, steam, or boil these foods rather than frying.
2. Place meat on a rack so the fat will drain off during cooking.
3. Use a nonstick spray and a nonstick pan to brown or fry foods.
4. Trim off visible fat before or after cooking.
5. If you add flour, bread crumbs, coating mixes, fat, or marinades when cooking, ask your dietitian how to count it in your meal plan.

VERY LEAN MEAT AND SUBSTITUTES LIST

One exchange equals 0 grams carbohydrate, 7 grams protein, 0–1 grams fat, and 35 calories.

One very lean meat exchange is equal to any one of the following items.

Poultry: Chicken or turkey (white meat, no skin), Cornish hen (no skin) . . . . .1 oz

Fish: Fresh or frozen cod, flounder, haddock, halibut, trout; tuna fresh or canned in water . . . . . . .1 oz

Shellfish: Clams, crab, lobster, scallops, shrimp, imitation shellfish . . . . .1 oz

Game: Duck or pheasant (no skin), venison, buffalo, ostrich . . . . .1 oz

Cheese with 1 gram or less fat per ounce:
Nonfat or low-fat cottage cheese . . . . .1/4 cup
Fat-free cheese . . . . .1 oz

Other: Processed sandwich meats with 1 gram or less fat per ounce, such as deli thin, shaved meats, chipped beef*, turkey ham . . . . 1 oz
Egg whites 2
Egg substitutes, plain . . . . .1/4 cup
Hot dogs with 1 gram or less fat per ounce . . . . . . .1 oz
Kidney (high in cholesterol) . . . . .1 oz
Sausage with 1 gram or less fat per ounce . . . . .1 oz

Count as one very lean meat and one starch exchange.

Dried beans, peas, lentils (cooked) . . . . .1/2 cup

LEAN MEAT AND SUBSTITUTES LIST

One exchange equals 0 grams carbohydrate, 7 grams protein, 3 grams fat, and 55 calories.

One lean meat exchange is equal to any one of the following items.

Beef: USDA Select or Choice grades of lean beef trimmed of fat, such as round, sirloin, and flank steak; tenderloin; roast (rib, chuck, rump); steak (T-bone, porterhouse, cubed), ground round . . . . .1 oz

Pork: Lean pork, such as fresh ham; canned, cured, or boiled ham; Canadian bacon*; tenderloin, center loin chop . . . . .1 oz

Lamb: Roast, chop, leg . . . . .1 oz

Veal: Lean chop, roast . . . . .1 oz

Poultry: Chicken, turkey (dark meat, no skin), chicken white meat (with skin), domestic duck or goose (well-drained of fat, no skin) . . . . .1 oz

Fish:
Herring (uncreamed or smoked) . . . . .1 oz
Oysters . . . . .6 medium
Salmon (fresh or canned), catfish . . . . .1 oz
Sardines (canned) . . . . .2 medium
Tuna (canned in oil, drained) . . . . .1 oz

Game: Goose (no skin), rabbit . . . . .1 oz

* = 400 mg or more of sodium per serving.

TABLE 8.2 Exchange Lists Summary Sheet *(Cont.)*

Lean Meats and Substitutes List Continued

Cheese:

4.5%-fat cottage cheese ....1/4 cup

Grated Parmesan ....2 Tbsp

Cheeses with 3 grams or less fat per ounce ....1 oz

Other:

Hot dogs with 3 grams or less fat per ounce* ... 1¹/₂ oz

Processed sandwich meat with 3 grams or less fat
per ounce, such as turkey pastrami or kielbasa .....1 oz

Liver, heart (high in cholesterol) ....1 oz

MEDIUM-FAT MEAT AND SUBSTITUTES LIST

One exchange equals 0 grams carbohydrate, 7 grams protein, 5 grams fat, and 75 calories.

One medium-fat meat exchange is equal to any one of the following items.

Beef: Most beef products fall into this category (ground beef, meatloaf, corned beef, short ribs, Prime grades of meat trimmed of fat, such as prime rib) ....1 oz

Pork: Top loin, chop, Boston butt, cutlet ....1 oz

Lamb: Rib roast, ground ....1 oz

Veal: Cutlet (ground or cubed, unbreaded) ....1 oz

Poultry: Chicken dark meat (with skin), ground turkey or ground chicken, fried chicken (with skin) ......1 oz

Fish: Any fried fish product ....1 oz

Cheese: With 5 grams or less fat per ounce

Feta ....1 oz

Mozzarella ....1 oz

Ricotta ....1/4 cup (2 oz)

Other:

Egg (high in cholesterol, limit to 3 per week) 1

Sausage with 5 grams or less fat per ounce ....1 oz

Soy milk ....1 cup

Tempeh ....1/4 cup

Tofu ....4 oz or 1/2 cup

HIGH-FAT MEAT AND SUBSTITUTES LIST

One exchange equals 0 grams carbohydrate, 7 grams protein, 8 grams fat, and 100 calories.

Remember these items are high in saturated fat, cholesterol, and calories and may raise blood cholesterol levels if eaten on a regular basis. One high-fat meat exchange is equal to any one of the following items.

Pork: Spareribs, ground pork, pork sausage ....1 oz

Cheese: All regular cheeses, such as American*, cheddar, Monterey Jack, Swiss ....1 oz

Other: Processed sandwich meats with 8 grams or less fat per ounce, such as bologna, pimento loaf, salami ..1 oz

Sausage, such as bratwurst, Italian, knockwurst, Polish, smoked ....1 oz

Hot dog (turkey or chicken)* 1 (10/lb)

* = 400 mg or more of sodium per serving.

Bacon ....3 slices (20 slices/lb)

Count as one high-fat meat plus one fat exchange.

Hot dog (beef, pork, or combination)* 1 (10/lb)

Peanut butter (contains unsaturated fat) ....2 Tbsp

FAT LIST

Fats are divided into three groups, based on the main type of fat they contain: monounsaturated, polyunsaturated, and saturated. Small amounts of monounsaturated and polyunsaturated fats in the foods we eat are linked with good health benefits. Saturated fats are linked with heart disease and cancer. In general, one fat exchange is:

• 1 teaspoon of regular margarine or vegetable oil,

• 1 tablespoon of regular salad dressings.

Nutrition Tips

1. All fats are high in calories. Limit serving sizes for good nutrition and health.

2. Nuts and seeds contain small amounts of fiber, protein, and magnesium.

3. If blood pressure is a concern, choose fats in the unsalted form to help lower sodium intake, such as unsalted peanuts.

Selection Tips

1. Check the Nutrition Facts on food labels for serving sizes. One fat exchange is based on a serving size containing 5 grams of fat.

2. When selecting regular margarine, choose those with liquid vegetable oil as the first ingredient. Soft margarines are not as saturated as stick margarines. Soft margarines are healthier choices. Avoid those listing hydrogenated or partially hydrogenated fat as the first ingredient.

3. When selecting low-fat margarines, look for liquid vegetable oil as the second ingredient. Water is usually the first ingredient.

4. When used in smaller amounts, bacon and peanut butter are counted as fat choices. When used in larger amounts, they are counted as high-fat meat choices.

5. Fat-free salad dressings are on the Other Carbohydrates list and the Free Foods list.

6. See the Free Foods list for nondairy coffee creamers, whipped topping, and fat-free products, such as margarines, salad dressings, mayonnaise, sour cream, cream cheese, and nonstick cooking spray.

MONOSATURATED FATS LIST

One fat exchange equals 5 grams fat and 45 calories.

Avocado, medium ....1/8 (1 oz)

Oil (canola, olive, peanut) ....1 tsp

Olives: ripe (black) ....8 large

TABLE 8.2 Exchange Lists Summary Sheet *(Cont.)*

Monosaturated Fats List Continued

green, stuffed* . . . . .10 large
Nuts
    almonds, cashews . . . . .6 nuts
    mixed (50% peanuts) . . . . .6 nuts
    peanuts . . . . .10 nuts
    pecans . . . . .4 halves
Peanut butter, smooth or crunchy . . . . .2 tsp
Sesame seeds . . . . .1 Tbsp
Tahini paste . . . . .2 tsp

POLYUNSATURATED FATS LIST

One fat exchange equals 5 grams fat and 45 calories.

Margarine: stick, tub, or squeeze . . . . .1 tsp
    lower-fat (30% to 50% vegetable oil) . . . . .1 Tbsp
Mayonnaise: regular . . . . .1 tsp
    reduced-fat . . . . .1 Tbsp
Nuts, walnuts, English . . . . .4 halves
Oil (corn, safflower, soybean) . . . . .1 tsp
Salad dressing: regular* . . . . .1 Tbsp
    reduced-fat . . . . .2 Tbsp
Miracle Whip Salad Dressing®: regular . . . . .2 tsp
    reduced-fat . . . . .1 Tbsp
Seeds: pumpkin, sunflower .1 Tbsp

SATURATED FATS LIST‡

One fat exchange equals 5 grams of fat and 45 calories.

Bacon, cooked . . . . .1 slice (20 slices/lb)
Bacon, grease . . . . .1 tsp
Butter: stick . . . . .1 tsp
    whipped . . . . .2 tsp
    reduced-fat . . . . .1 Tbsp
Chitterlings, boiled . . . . .2 Tbsp (1/2 oz)
Coconut, sweetened, shredded . . . . .2 Tbsp
Cream, half and half . . . . .2 Tbsp
Cream cheese: regular . . . . .1 Tbsp (1/2 oz)
    reduced-fat . . . . .2 Tbsp (1 oz)
Fatback or salt pork, see below†
Shortening or lard . . . . .1 tsp
Sour cream: regular . . . . .2 Tbsp
    reduced-fat . . . . .3 Tbsp

†Use a piece 1 in. × 1 in. × 1/4 in. if you plan to eat the fatback cooked with vegetables. Use a piece 2 in. × 1 in. × 1/2 in. when eating only the vegetables with the fatback removed.

‡ Saturated fats can raise blood cholesterol levels.

FREE FOODS LIST

A *free food* is any food or drink that contains less than 20 calories or less than 5 grams of carbohydrate per serving. Foods with a serving size listed should be limited to three servings per day. Foods listed without a serving size can be eaten as often as you like.

Fat-free Or Reduced-fat Foods

Cream cheese, fat-free . . . . .1 Tbsp
Creamers, nondairy, liquid . . . . .1 Tbsp
Creamers, nondairy, powdered . . . . .2 tsp
Mayonnaise, fat-free . . . . .1 Tbsp
Mayonnaise, reduced-fat . . . . .1 tsp
Margarine, fat-free . . . . .4 Tbsp
Margarine, reduced-fat . . . . .1 tsp
Miracle Whip®, nonfat . . . . .1 Tbsp
Miracle Whip®, reduced-fat . . . . .1 tsp
Nonstick cooking spray
Salad dressing, fat-free . . . . .1 Tbsp
Salad dressing, fat-free, Italian . . . . .2 Tbsp
Salsa . . . . .1/4 cup
Sour cream, fat-free, reduced-fat . . . . .1 Tbsp
Whipped topping, regular or light . . . . .2 Tbsp

Sugar-free Or Low-sugar Foods

Candy, hard, sugar-free . . . . .1 candy
Gelatin dessert, sugar-free
Gelatin, unflavored
Gum, sugar-free
Jam or jelly, low-sugar or light . . . . .2 tsp
Sugar substitutes§
Syrup, sugar-free . . . . .2 Tbsp

§Sugar substitutes, alternatives, or replacements that are approved by the Food and Drug Administration (FDA) are safe to use. Common brand names include:

    Equal® (as (aspartame)

    Sprinkle Sweet® (saccharin)

    Sweet One® (acesulfame K)

    Sweet-10® (saccharin)

    Sugar Twin® (saccharin)

    Sweet'n Low® (saccharin)

Drinks

Bouillon, broth, consommé*
Bouillon or broth, low-sodium
Carbonated or mineral water
Cocoa powder, unsweetened . . . . .1 Tbsp
Coffee
Club soda
Diet soft drinks, sugar-free
Drink mixes, sugar-free
Tea
Tonic water, sugar-free

Condiments

Catsup . . . . .1 Tbsp
Horseradish
Lemon juice
Lime juice
Mustard
Pickles, dill* . . . . .1½ large
Soy sauce, regular or light*
Taco sauce . . . . .1 Tbsp
Vinegar

TABLE 8.2 Exchange Lists Summary Sheet *(Cont.)*

Seasonings

Be careful with seasonings that contain sodium or are salts, such as garlic or celery salt, and lemon pepper.

Flavoring extracts

Garlic

Herbs, fresh or dried

Pimento

Spices

Tabasco® or hot pepper sauce

Wine, used in cooking

Worcestershire sauce

COMBINATION FOODS LIST

Many of the foods we eat are mixed together in various combinations. These combination foods do not fit into any one exchange list. Often it is hard to tell what is in a casserole dish or prepared food item. This is a list of exchanges for some typical combination foods. This list will help you fit these foods into your meal plan. Ask your dietitian for information about any other combination foods you would like to eat.

Food	Serving Size	Exchanges Per Serving
Entrees		
Tuna noodle casserole, lasagna, spaghetti with meatballs, chili with beans, macaroni and cheese*	1 cup (8 oz)	2 carbohydrates, 2 medium-fat meats
Chow mein (without noodles or rice)*	2 cups (16 oz)	1 carbohydrate, 2 lean meats
Pizza, cheese, thin crust*	1/4 of 10 in. (5 oz)	2 carbohydrates, 2 medium-fat meats, 1 fat
Pizza, meat topping, thin crust*	1/4 of 10 in. (5 oz)	2 carbohydrates, 2 medium-fat meats, 2 fats
Pot pie*	1 (7 oz)	2 carbohydrates, 1 medium-fat meat, 4 fats
Frozen entrees		
Salisbury steak with gravy, mashed potato*	1 (11 oz)	2 carbohydrates, 3 medium-fat meats, 3-4 fats
Turkey with gravy, mashed potato, dressing*	1 (11 oz)	2 carbohydrates, 2 medium-fat meats, 2 fats
Entree with less than 300 calories*	1 (8 oz)	2 carbohydrates, 3 lean meats
Soups		
Bean*	1 cup	1 carbohydrate, 1 very lean meat
Cream (made with water)*	1 cup (8 oz)	1 carbohydrate, 1 fat
Split pea (made with water)*	1/2 cup (4 oz)	1 carbohydrate
Tomato (made with water)*	1 cup (8 oz)	1 carbohydrate
Vegetable beef, chicken noodle or other broth-type*	1 cup (8 oz)	1 carbohydrate
Burritos with beef*	2	4 carbohydrates, 2 medium-fat meats, 2 fats
Chicken nuggets*	6	1 carbohydrate, 2 medium-fat meats, 1 fat
Chicken breast and wing, breaded and fried*	1 each	1 carbohydrate, 4 medium-fat meats, 2 fats
Fish sandwich/tartar sauce*	1	3 carbohydrates, 1 medium-fat meat, 3 fats
French fries, thin	20–25	2 carbohydrates, 2 fats
Hamburger, regular	1	2 carbohydrates, 2 medium-fat meats
Hamburger, large*	1	2 carbohydrates, 3 medium-fat meats, 1 fat
Hot dog with bun*	1	1 carbohydrate, 1 high-fat meat, 1 fat
Individual pan pizza*	1	5 carbohydrates, 3 medium-fat meats, 3 fats
Soft-serve cone	1 medium	2 carbohydrates, 1 fat
Submarine sandwich*	1 sub (6 in)	3 carbohydrates, 1 vegetable, 2 medium-fat meats, 1 fat
Taco, hard shell*	1 (6 oz)	2 carbohydrates, 2 medium-fat meats, 2 fats
Taco, soft shell*	1 (3 oz)	1 carbohydrate, 1 medium-fat meat, 1 fat

Ask at your fast-food restaurant for nutrition information about your favorite fast foods.

* = 400 mg or more of sodium per serving.

by 4 calories per gram, and fat calories by 9 calories per gram.

4. Translate grams of protein, carbohydrate, and fat into exchanges from the food list. Pick the number of servings from each exchange group according to individual food preferences and usual diet. Add up grams of proteins, carbohydrates, and fats from each exchange group and adjust number of servings as needed to approximate desired grams of proteins, carbohydrates, and fats.

5. Distribute the servings from all the exchanges lists into meals and snacks based on the individual's usual dietary habits. Individuals taking insulin will need to have their exchanges distributed to match their insulin schedules as well as food preferences.

SAMPLE MEAL PLANS

Sample 1,200-calorie meal plan

Let's say, for example, you are designing a meal plan for an inactive middle-age female who weighs 170 pounds.

1. **Estimate energy needs:** An estimate of her calorie needs to maintain weight would be 170 pounds × 10 calories per pound = 1,700 calories. To lose about a pound weekly, you subtract out 500 calories daily, leaving a calorie level for weight loss of 1,200 calories daily. (You will also help the patient work out an exercise plan, which should help her to lose more than a pound weekly.)

2. **Distribute calories:**

Carbohydrate: 0.55 × 1,200 calories = 660 calories

Protein: 0.20 × 1,200 calories = 240 calories

Fat: 0.25 × 1,200 calories = 300 calories

3. **Convert calories to grams:**

660 calories/4 calories per gram = 165 grams of carbohydrate

TABLE 8.3 Nutrient Content of Exchange Groups

Groups/List	Carbohydrate (grams)	Protein (grams)	Fat (grams)	Calories
Carbohydrate Group				
Starch	15	3	1 or less	80
Fruit	15	–	–	60
Milk				
Skim	12	8	0–3	90
Low-fat	12	8	5	120
Whole	12	8	8	150
Other carbohydrates	15	varies	varies	varies
Vegetables	5	2	–	25
Meat and Meat Substitute Group				
Very lean	–	7	0–1	35
Lean	–	7	3	55
Medium-fat	–	7	5	75
High-fat	–	7	8	100
Fat Group	–	–	5	45

Source: American Diabetes and Dietetic Associations. (1996). *Exchange Lists for Weight Management.* Alexandria, VA: The American Diabetes Association, Chicago, Il: The American Dietetic Association.

60 calories/4 calories per gram = 60 grams of protein

300 calories/9 calories per gram = 33 grams of fat

4. **Translate grams into exchanges:**

When translating grams of nutrients into exchange groups, keep the individual's usual dietary pattern in mind. The greater the calorie level of the diet, the more flexibility you have in planning the exchanges. The following meal plan would provide approximately the desired calories and grams of carbohydrates, proteins, and fats

6 starch exchanges

4 lean or very lean meat exchanges

3 vegetable exchanges

2 fruit exchanges

2 skim milk exchanges

3 fat exchanges

5. **Distribute exchanges into meals and snacks.**

Again, it is helpful to base distribution of

exchanges on the individual's usual eating pattern, unless the patient must follow a more rigid meal pattern because of insulin or other medication use. If a patient is used to having several snacks daily, then plan them in to the meal pattern. However, try to avoid consuming the bulk of the exchanges late in the day. It is also helpful to give patients a sample menu as an example:

Breakfast:

2 starch exchanges	1 ounce ready-to-eat cereal
	1 slice whole-grain toast
1 fat exchange	1 teaspoon margarine
1 milk exchange	1 cup skim milk
1 fruit exchange	1/2 grapefruit

Lunch:

2 starch exchanges	2 slices pumpernickel bread
1 meat exchange	1 ounce sliced turkey
1 fat exchange	1 tablespoon reduced-calorie mayonnaise
free food	lettuce
1 fruit exchange	1¼ cup whole strawberries
1 vegetable exchange	1 cup raw carrot sticks
free food	Decaffeinated coffee

Supper:

3 meat exchanges	6 ounces boiled shrimp
1 starch exchange	1 small baked potato
2 vegetable exchanges	1 cup cooked broccoli
1 fat exchange	1 teaspoon margarine
free food	Decaffeinated coffee

Snack:

1 milk exchange	8 ounces plain nonfat yogurt
1 "other" carbohydrate	
substituted for starch	
exchange	1 fat-free cookie

Sample 1,800-calorie meal plan

Following the same steps as listed previously, this sample 1,800-calorie meal plan was developed:

9 starch exchanges

3 lean or very lean meat exchanges

3 medium-fat meat exchanges

3 vegetable exchanges

3 fruit exchanges

2 skim milk exchanges

5 fat exchanges

As the calorie level of the diet increases, the more freedom the individual has to substitute foods from the "other" carbohydrate list for starch, fruit, or milk exchanges. Patient and therapist should keep in mind, however, that nutrient content of these foods are generally not as high as foods in the other groups. In addition, because many of these foods are concentrated sources of calories, they may not be as filling as foods in the starch, fruit, or milk group.

BEHAVIOR MODIFICATION STRATEGIES

Behavior modification programs for weight control are designed to make the individual aware of eating behaviors that promote obesity and help them gradually change these behaviors and the eating environment to promote weight loss or maintenance. While behavior modification by itself produces only modest weight losses, the effectiveness of behavior modification is enhanced by combining it with dietary restriction or more aggressive approaches such as very low-calorie diets or drug therapy for obesity (Wilson, 1995). Likewise the effectiveness of diet approaches is enhanced by adding a behavior modification component, since behavior change is considered integral to long-term weight maintenance.

Target behaviors that require change for many

obese individuals are eating and exercise habits. To change behaviors, current behaviors must first be assessed.

Keeping a Food Diary

Instructing patients to keep a daily food diary by recording food intake and circumstances under which food was eaten greatly increases understanding of the patient's food habits and usually improves adherence to recommended diet changes. Physical activity can also be included on the food diary or recorded on a separate diary.

The diet diary can be reviewed at each clinic visit, providing a teaching tool. Keeping a daily food diary accomplishes several goals

- Increases awareness of food intake

- Provides a teaching tool to learn about aspects of the diet or calorie content of foods

- Helps patients and counselors learn about eating patterns and relationship of eating to other events or feelings

- Fosters control over eating

- Provides a written record of calories, which can be related to weight change

Figure 8.1 shows a sample of a very detailed food diary, where the patient records not only type and amount of food eaten, but also the time the patient started and stopped eating, the place, the physical position, who the patient was with and what the patient was doing while eating, the patient's mood, the patient's hunger level at the time, and whether the food was considered a meal or snack.

Detailed diaries such as these can help patients and counselors learn about behaviors, emotions, and activities that promote overeating and weight gain. However, it is not always necessary for patient to keep such detailed diaries. Even a simple record of food or drink and amount scratched daily on a pocket notebook will greatly increase patient awareness of eating habits and improve diet adherence.

For the greatest effectiveness, patients should be instructed to record *everything* they eat or drink, except for water. They should record this right after eating, not later that evening or the next day. To do this, food diaries should be carried with the patient wherever he or she goes.

Setting Realistic Goals

Goals of behavior modification are different from weight loss goals—they are behavioral steps intended to gradually shape eating or exercise behavior or the eating environment, which will, in turn, influence body weight. A good behavioral goal must be individualized, specific, realistic, and designed to help control unhelpful eating behavior. Examples of specific, realistic goals include

- To reduce candy bar consumption, I will eat a piece of fruit for a snack during my afternoon break three times this week.

- To reduce overeating when I'm depressed, the next time I'm depressed in the evening I will take a half-hour walk.

- I will have one scoop of frozen low-fat yogurt or fruit rather than a heavy dessert after dinner three times this week.

Designing Tactics

Individualized tactics are then designed to help the individual modify the eating environment and eating and exercise behavior. For example, if analysis of the food diary shows that the individual eats in many rooms of the home or particularly in the room where the television is, a tactic might be to only eat in one room of the house, for example, the kitchen or dining room.

If the individual tastes food while cooking or clearing the table, a tactic might be to have someone else do the dishes or to sit down while eating to increase awareness of eating. If coffee breaks at work pose a eating problem, a tactic might be to walk stairs during break instead of going into the coffee room.

FIGURE 8.1 Sample Food Diary

Date________________________Name ____

Time												
Start	End	Place	Phy Pos	Alone or with whom	Assoc. Activity	M	H	M/S	Amount	Food or Beverage	Calories
6–11											
11–4											
4–9											
9–6											

Percent of entries filled out right before or after eating 0 25 50 75 100 [ ]

Source: Henry A. Jordan, Leonard S. Levitz, and Gordon M. Kimbrell, "Food Intake Record" from *Eating is Okay.* Copyright© 1976 by Associates for Behaviors Education and S & R Gelman Associates Inc. Reprinted with permission of Rawson Associates; an imprint of Macmillian Publishing Company.

Table 8.4 lists some possible tactics to help modify eating and exercise behavior and the eating environment.

Reinforcing Behavior Change

A reinforcer is anything that occurs during or follows a behavior that increases the likelihood that a particular behavior will occur again in the future. Reinforcers can be positive or negative. Negative reinforcers are what motivate many people to join weight control programs—fear of weight-related diseases, failure of a relationship, feeling tired of having clothes not fit, or feeling out-of-shape. Examples of positive reinforcement include having clothes fit more loosely, enjoying compliments from others, freedom from joint pain, job advancement, informal blood sugar levels, or feeling more energetic.

TABLE 8.4 Tactic Summary List

NUTRITION TACTICS

Tactics for choosing and preparing food:
Shop from a list based on healthy meal plans
Read food labels to select low-fat, fiber-rich foods
Bake, broil, or grill instead of fry or saute in fat
Shop when not hungry
Sip water while preparing food to avoid sampling
Calculate percentage calories from fat in foods

Tactics for environment and eating style:
Take at least 20 minutes to eat my meal
Do nothing else but converse while eating
Eat at least three times throughout the day
Plan for snacks
Sit down at the dining room table to eat
Drink a glass of water before a meal
Store food out of sight
Ask someone else to clean up the leftovers
Substitute herbs and spices for salt
Enter the house through a different door
Take a different route

Tactics for eating out:
Ask to have problem foods left off the plate
Immediately portion out what to eat, leave the rest to take home
Eat a low-calorie snack before going out
Plan my meal selection before going out
Ask that food be prepared without added fat (broiled, baked, or grilled)
Ask for dressings, sauces, and toppings on the side
Avoid alcohol

Physical activity tactics:
Daily stretching exercises
Aerobic exercise_____days per week for_____minutes

Keep a weekly exercise diary
Try a new activity I was too out of shape to do in the past
Play active games with my children
Take the stairs rather than the elevator
Park and walk from the far side of the parking lot
Ride my bike to work
Invite a friend to exercise with me

Stress and time management tactics:
Practice relaxation using cassette tapes
Write a plan for a project I've been avoiding
Use behavioral rehearsal before a trouble-prone situation
Work off stress hormones with exercise
Go for a walk instead of cooking when angry or anxious

Social support:
Ask for support and encouragement from family and friends
Express appreciation to family and friends
Exercise with a friend or a group

Beliefs, attitudes, thoughts, and body image:
Practice stopping negative thoughts and replacing them with more useful thoughts
Use behavioral rehearsal of new thought patterns before a trouble-prone situation
Focus on gradual lifestyle changes instead of dieting or weight loss
Accept compliments graciously
Look in the mirror daily and remind myself, "I am making choices for health and well-being...because I'm worth it."
When faced with unhealthy foods, ask myself, "Do I really want it?" instead of "Should I have it, do I need it, and can I get away with it?"

In behavior modification, individuals and therapists try to positively reinforce new behaviors and goals achieved. Positive reinforcement, or rewards, can be linked to the patient's goals and tactics to help them reach their goals. Examples of positive rewards include buying a new piece of clothing in a smaller size, taking a long, relaxing bath, attending a play or concert, taking a weekend trip, or adding money to a jar to be used for a bigger reward in the future.

Family, friends, and support can also provide the patient with positive reinforcement and help them maintain new habits over the long-term. Enlisting the help and support of significant others will help the patient maintain positive behavior changes over the long-term.

NUTRITION COUNSELING STRATEGIES

For nutrition counseling to be most effective, nutrition counselors should

- Create a good setting
- Build rapport with good communication
- Listen carefully
- Avoid yes or no questions
- Help the patient identify and plan goals
- Give frequent feedback
- Be specific about what is expected
- Encourage family involvement
- Be supportive

The National Heart, Lung and Blood Institute (1991) gives eight tips to help improve patient adherence to nutrition plans

Relate—If nurses can relate well with their patients and develop a close and caring relationship, the patient will be more likely to adhere to advice given.

Communicate—Be clear in what you are trying to say. Give specific advice, repeat it, and ask the patient to repeat it to be certain they understand what you are trying to say.

Motivate—Increase motivation by breaking dietary change into small but progressive steps and setting realistic short-term goals.

Educate—Use or develop educational aids to help patients understand their current eating patterns and the desired eating patterns.

Collaborate—Encourage support from the patient's family and refer the patient to other professionals or self-help or support groups as needed.

Facilitate—Make dietary changes easier by making changes gradually. Keep changes as simple as possible.

Innovate—Use innovative methods to increase adherence, such as giving token rewards for short-term goals achieved, having patients contribute their favorite healthy recipes, or creating a lending library of related health or cookbooks.

Calculate—Keep track of the success of your patients in reaching dietary and exercise. Note improvements in blood pressure, blood cholesterol levels, blood sugar levels and other risk factors for chronic diseases.

The next chapter describes aggressive approaches to obesity management for individuals with severe obesity, obesity-related health risks, and individuals who have been unsuccessful with conservative approaches.

EXAM QUESTIONS

CHAPTER 8
Questions 54–60

54. The two main considerations in evaluating commercial and popular diets should be

    a. effectiveness and cost

    b. location and cost

    c. safety and effectiveness

    d. safety and personnel

55. Based on the Food Exchange Lists, a baked potato would belong in which list?

    a. starch list

    b. vegetable list

    c. fruit list

    d. other carbohydrates list

56. Based on the Food Exchange Lists, peanut butter would belong in which list?

    a. high-fat meat and meat substitute list

    b. medium-fat meat and meat substitute list

    c. starch list

    d. fat list

57. How many grams of carbohydrates does one exchange from the starch list provide?

    a. 5

    b. 10

    c. 15

    d. 20

58. The first step in calculating meal plans based on the food exchange lists is to

    a. distribute calories into desired percentages of proteins, carbohydrates, and fats

    b. convert calories from proteins, carbohydrates, and fats into grams

    c. translate grams of proteins, carbohydrates, and fats into exchanges from the food list

    d. estimate energy needs

59. Helpful behavior modification strategies include which of the following?

    a. making food behavior charts while eating

    b. keeping a food diary

    c. setting a large reward for reaching ideal body weight

    d. sticking to a 1,200-calorie diet

60. Patient adherence to nutrition plans can be improved by which of the following?

    a. education

    b. communication

    c. motivation

    d. all of the above

CHAPTER 9

INTERVENTION: AGGRESSIVE MANAGEMENT OF OBESITY

CHAPTER OBJECTIVE

After reading this chapter, you will be able to describe the types of aggressive interventions used for management of obesity.

LEARNING OBJECTIVES

After studying this chapter, you will be able to

1. Recognize patients who are candidates for aggressive intervention for obesity.

2. Identify characteristics of low and very low-calorie diets and recommendations for use.

3. Indicate when drug therapy is appropriate for obesity management and specify components of therapy.

4. Specify types of surgeries used in the management of obesity.

INTRODUCTION

Aggressive obesity interventions include low-calorie diets of 800 to 1,200 calories daily, very low-calorie diet programs of 500 to 800 calories daily, use of antiobesity drugs, and gastric surgery. Aggressive obesity interventions should be undertaken only under close medical supervision and for limited periods of time. Most sound aggressive interventions are clinic- or hospital-based programs involving a multidiscipli-nary team of nurses, physicians, dietitians, exercise physiologists, psychologists, and health educators.

This chapter will review the types of aggressive management approaches used in obesity intervention.

WHO IS AGGRESSIVE INTERVENTION APPROPRIATE FOR?

Aggressive management approaches for obesity are usually reserved for individuals with severe obesity (>100 percent over ideal body weight, or a BMI of >35). Individuals with moderate levels of obesity (40 to 100 percent over ideal, or a BMI of 30 to 35), and other obesity-related health risks—such as high blood pressure, high blood lipid levels, or non-insulin-dependent diabetes—may also be candidates for aggressive intervention.

Although these are general guidelines, the physician and nurse must evaluate each patient individually, considering relevant factors such as age, motivation, medical risk, and past weight loss attempts. Patients who pursue aggressive approaches to obesity treatment can also benefit from techniques used in conservative management as they strive to maintain weight loss over the long-term. For example, a 12-week phase of very low-calorie dieting might be followed by a

1,500-calorie balanced-deficit diet using the exchange lists and behavior modification tactics to help prevent regaining of weight-lost.

As with all weight-loss approaches, increasing physical activity should be a part of aggressive management approaches. Patients who are older, severely obese, or have related health risks should increase physical activity only under the guidance of their physician, as discussed in chapter twelve. They may also need to consult an exercise physiologist for help in designing an individualized physical activity regimen.

LOW-CALORIE DIETS

Low-calorie diets are definedas providing 800 to 1,200 calories daily and should be used only with proper physician approval, medical screening, and close medical supervision (Food and Nutrition Board, 1995). Levels of medications may need to be adjusted or decreased during the course of low-calorie diet therapy.

Some low-calorie diets use regular foods, while others use special formulas or supplements. Commercial diet programs that offer a low-calorie component of their program include Weight Watchers, Diet Workshop, Diet Center Jenny Craig, and Nutri\System (Food and Nutrition Board, 1995). Low-calorie diet products include Sweet Success (Nestle) and Slim Fast. While these specially formulated diet products can produce weight losses, using them without medical supervision is not advised. Further, special formulas do not teach patients how to make food choices in a real-life eating environment.

Low-calorie diets can also be designed using the food exchange lists described in chapter 8 and shown in *Tables 8.2 and 8.3.* Low-calorie diets using regular foods require supplementation with a low-dose multivitamin and mineral preparation. No matter how nutritious patients' food choices are, it is almost impossible to achieve adequate vitamin and mineral intake when consuming only 800 to 1,000 calories daily.

The lower the calorie content of the diet, the lower the percentage of calories from fat should be. Low-calorie diets usually contain no more than 25 percent of calories as fat and should provide 0.8 to 1.5 grams of protein per kilogram of body weight. The sample 1,000-calorie meal plan shown below and based on the exchange lists provides about 24 percent of calories as proteins, 20 percent as fats, and 56 percent as carbohydrates. To design other low-calorie meal patterns based on the exchange lists, see the section "Steps in Calculating a Meal Plan" in chapter eight.

Sample 1,000-Calorie Meal Plan

5 starch exchanges

4 very lean meat exchanges

3 vegetable exchanges

2 fruit exchanges

2 skim milk exchanges

2 fat exchanges

A sample menu based on the above meal plan is shown below:

Breakfast:

1 starch exchange	1/2 cup shredded wheat cereal
1 fruit exchange	3/4 cup blueberries
1 skim milk exchange	1 cup skim milk

Lunch:

1 starch exchange	4 slices melba toast
2 vegetable exchanges	2 cups salad greens
free food	1t fat-free dressing
1 very lean meat exchange	1 ounce turkey ham
1 fruit exchange	1 medium fresh peach

Supper:

3 very lean meat exchanges	3 ounces baked skinless chicken
1 vegetable exchange	1/2 cup steamed broccoli
2 starches exchanges	1 small baked potato
	1 small whole wheat roll
1 skim milk exchange	1 cup plain nonfat yogurt
1 fat exchange	1 teaspoon margarine

Snack:

1 starch exchange	2 rice cakes
1 fat exchange	2 teaspoons peanut butter

VERY LOW-CALORIE DIETS

Very low-calorie diets (VLCD) were first developed to help prevent the dangerous and sometimes lethal loss of lean body mass with total fasting. However, several deaths occurred on VLCD using liquid protein in the mid to late 1970s (Lantingua, 1980).

In the 1980s very low-calorie diets (VLCD) again became popular as a means of achieving large weight losses over relatively short time periods (Wadden, 1983). The VLCD of the 1980s differed from the early ones in that they provided high-quality proteins and adequate amounts of vitamins and minerals. Use of VLCD has decreased in the 1990s with the rise in antidieting sentiment (Wadden, 1995).

The VLCD of today usually provide

- 500 to 800 calories daily, or about six to 10 calories per kilogram of body weight

- 1.2 to 1.5 grams of high-quality proteins per kilogram of ideal body weight

- 30 to 45 grams of carbohydrate

- 2 to 5 grams of fat

- 100 percent of the recommended allowance for essential vitamins and minerals

- 2 liters of noncaloric fluid (Wadden, 1995)

Initial weight losses on VLCD are usually rapid, partly due to sodium and water losses. Thereafter weight losses on VLCD can average two to four pounds weekly. Because of the low-calorie level, most of the calories on VLCD come from high-quality proteins to help preserve lean body mass. Protein can be provided from food or from a liquid supplement (Perri, 1992). VLCD based on food are also called protein-sparing modified fasts (PSMF) and usually provide 1.5 grams of protein per kilogram of ideal body weight. Protein is derived from lean meats, fish, and poultry supplemented with vitamins, minerals, and electrolytes.

With liquid VLCD, protein is usually derived from a milk-, soy-, or egg-based powder that is mixed with water and consumed three to five or more times daily. Vitamins, minerals, and electrolytes are sometimes included in the formula or sometimes taken separately. A small amount of carbohydrates is also provided to help minimize water losses and electrolyte abnormalities. Example of commercial VLCD programs using such formulas include Optifast, Medifast, New Directions, and Health Management Resources (HMR). The advantage of formula-based VLCD are that they eliminate choice and promote patient adherence. VLCD are usually administered in three phases

1. The VLCD phase, lasting 12 to 16 weeks

2. The refeeding phase, lasting 4 to 6 weeks

3. The maintenance phase, lasting 4 to 8 weeks or longer

VLCD are appropriate only for patients with severe obesity or moderate obesity and obesity-related risk factors who have tried more conservative approaches to weight loss. Contraindications to a VLCD include recent heart disease, stroke, cancer type I diabetes, liver or renal failure, or severe psychological disorders (Perri, 1992). Side effects of VLCD can include headaches, fatigue, hypotension, constipation, gallbladder disease, and menstrual irregularity (Atkinson, 1989). VLCD are also expensive, often costing $2,500 or more for 20 weeks of treatment.

VLCD are considered relatively safe when used appropriately. According to Perri (1992), appropriate use includes

1. Complete medical screening prior to entry in the program

2. Exclusion of patients with mild obesity or contraindications

3. Weekly or biweekly medical supervision while on the program, including during the refeeding phase

4. Limit of 12 weeks on the VLCD phase

5. Routine blood tests and electrocardiograms to evaluate electrolyte balance and cardiac functioning, and

6. Instruction and follow-up during the weight maintenance phase

While VLCD yield impressive weight losses, long-term results are still discouraging. Although patients on VLCD lost more weight during treatment compared to patients on balanced-deficit diets, patients on VLCD had regained a substantial portion of the weight they had lost and had body weights comparable to those treated with more conservative deficit diets by $1\frac{1}{2}$ years after treatment.

Combining behavior modification with VLCD may improve results slightly. Wadden and colleagues (1989) studied weight losses five years after initial treatment with either a VLCD, behavior modification, or a combination of both. Initially weight losses were greatest with the combined therapy. At the end of five years, however, the majority of participants from all three treatment

groups had regained all the weight initially lost. Eleven percent of subjects in the VLCD-alone group, 13 percent of subjects in the behavior modification group, and 27 percent of subjects in the combined VLCD plus behavior modification group maintained losses of 11 pounds or more at the five-year follow-up.

PHARMACOLOGICAL INTERVENTION

In the past, regulations in most states prohibited prescribing an antiobesity drug for longer than three months. The common belief was that anti-obesity drugs should be used only for short periods of time, usually 12–16 weeks, to correct metabolic imbalances (Guy-Grand, 1992). Once the obese person had lost weight, the antiobesity drug could be discontinued. Since most obese individuals regained weight lost, drug therapy was viewed as ineffective and discouraged.

Many groups have claimed the standards used to evaluate antiobesity drugs are unreasonable (Food and Nutrition Board, 1995). The current belief is that obesity is a chronic disease requiring long-term management. Just as some individuals with hypertension or non-insulin-dependent diabetes benefit from long-term drug therapy, so might some obese individuals.

Antiobesity drugs fall into two categories (Heshka and Heymsfield, 1995)

1. Agents that reduce net energy intake

2. Agents that increase net energy expenditure

Of those that reduce net energy intake, some reduce the level of hunger, while others increase satiety. Appetite suppressant drugs include the amphetamines, which have a high potential for addiction and are now rarely used. Another class of drugs suppress appetite but have greatly reduced stimulatory action on the central nervous system and a low abuse potential compared to amphetamines. These drugs include

- Phentermine (hydrochloride and resin)

- Phenmetrazine (hydrochloride)

- Phendimetrazine (tartrate)

- Diethylpropion (hydrochloride)

- Mazindol

- Phenylpropanolamine

Another group of drugs decrease net energy intake by altering serotonergic pathways. These include

- Fluoxetine

- Sibutramine

Other medications interfere with nutrient absorption in the gastrointestinal tract and increase energy losses in the feces. One such agent is tetrahydrolipstatin, which interferes with fat absorption. However, such agents can cause unacceptable side effects for some individuals.

Of the agents that increase energy expenditure, most also affect cardiac function. For example, thyroid hormone should not be prescribed during dieting because it can increase loss of body protein, including cardiac tissue. Ephedrine is currently the only available drug in this category that increases energy expenditure without affecting cardiac function (Heshka and Heymsfield, 1995).

Guidelines for pharmacological intervention for obesity include

- Use only for patients with a BMI >30 or a BMI >27 if other risk factors are present.

- Use only in patients who have tried other weight-loss approaches.

- Patients should have a thorough physical examination and regular medical monitoring during use.

- Combine pharmacological intervention with dietary instruction and increased physical activity.

Factors to be considered in selecting a drug include (Guy-Grand, 1992)

- Clinical tolerance

- Absence of addictive properties

- Sustained effects over the long-term

- Absence of major side effects and hazards

- Known mechanism of action

FENFLURAMINE AND DEXFENFLURAMINE

Two antiobesity drugs were widely used in 1996 and 1997 for obesity management. Fenfluramine and dexfenfluramine helped decreased net energy intake by altering serotonin metabolism in the body, increasing serotonin activity int he brain and reducing appetite.

However, these two drugs were withdrawn by their manufacturers in September of 1997 because of potentially serious heart valve damage and increased risk of primary pulmonary hypertension, a rare but often fatal disorder that destroys blood vessels in the heart and lungs.

Background

In April of 1996, the Food and Drug Administration (FDA) approved the first new antiobesity drug for use in the United States in 23 years: dexfenfluramine. Dexfenfluramine was manufactured for Interneuron Pharmaceuticals and marketed under the name of Redux by Wyeth-Ayerst Laboratories, a subsidiary of American Home Products Corp., Madison, NJ. Dexfenfluramine was intended to aid in the management of obesity by increasing serotonin levels in the brain and reducing appetite.

A related drug, fenfluramine had been approved for use in the Unites States by the FDA several years earlier. Fenfluramine, manufactured and marketed under the name Pondimin by Wyeth-Ayerst Laboratories, contains a mix of both levofenfluramine and dexfenfluramine, which are mirror images of each other. Although levofenfluramine and fenfluramine both cause drowsiness, dexfenfluramine does not.

In 1992, scientists discovered that using fenfluramine in combination with the mild amphetamine-like drug phentermine caused little drowsiness and effectively suppressed appetite. Use of the fenfluramine-phentermine combination, nicknamed fen-phen, increased rapidly during the next few years. Although the FDA had approved each of these drugs for use separately, use of the drugs in combination was never approved.

Fueled by the approval of dexfenfluramine, interest in antiobesity drugs skyrocketed in 1996 and 1997. In 1996 alone, the total number of prescriptions for the fen-phen combination exceeded 18 million. Many prescriptions for these antiobesity drugs were written by physicians with no special experience or training in weight management.

Health Concerns

A serious outbreak of primary pulmonary hypertension occurred in Europe between 1967 and 1972 that was eventually linked to the appetite suppressant drug aminorex. The drug was then recalled from the market, but not before hundreds of people were seriously affected (Follath et al., 1971). More recently, use of dexfenfluramine and fenfluramine in Europe led to more cases of primary pulmonary hypertension (McMurray et al., 1986).

In 1997, data from the United States began to emerge that suggested that not only were the risks of primary pulmonary hypertension greater than expected, but that use of these drugs was associated with heart valve damage. Doctors at Mayo Clinic in Rochester, MN, and at MeritCare Medical Center in Fargo, ND, first determined that heart valve problems were associated with the use of fen-phen. A review of 24 patients who had taken fen-phen for 1 to 28 months and who had no history of heart disease showed that all 24 women were shown to have significant heart valve damage as assessed by echocardiography, a special procedure that can test the functioning of heart valves (Connolly et al., 1997). The damaged heart valves were thickened, causing blood to flow backward, or leak, through the valve. This leaking action causes the heart to work harder and can lead to congestive heart failure. Open-heart surgery to was required for 5 of the patients. One third of the 24 women also had primary pulmonary hypertension.

These findings prompted the FDA to request that physicians across the country report any similar findings. Follow-up results were dramatic, with records of 291 patients from five other medical centers indicating that about 30% of patients taking either dexfenfluramine or fen-phen had abnormal findings on echocardiograms even though the patients had no signs or symptoms. The echocardiograms of these patients revealed heart valve damage similar to the type seen in the Mayo Clinic study. Some of these patients also required open-heart surgery to repair damaged valves.

Additional cases of primary pulmonary hypertension and heart valve damage associated with use of both dexfenfluramine and fenfluramine were also reported (Cannistra, Davis, & Bauman, 1997; Curfman, 1997; Graham & Green, 1997). One investigator reported a case of fatal primary pulmonary hypertension in a woman who had taken fen-phen for just 23 days (Mark Patalas, Chang, Evans, & Kessler, 1997).

These findings prompted the FDA to request that manufacturers withdraw fenfluramine and dexfenfluramine from the market. In September of 1997, manufacturers voluntarily withdrew these two drugs. Phentermine, the second half of the fen-phen combination, was not associated with heart valve problems and is still available, although it can no longer be used with fenfluramine.

Recommendations

Persons who had taken fenfluramine or dexfenfluramine either alone or in combination with phentermine were advised in September of 1997 to talk with their doctor and discontinue these drugs. A gradual tapering off of the drugs was generally recommended, because abrupt withdrawal could increase risk of depression.

Reports of pulmonary hypertension and valvular damage associated with use of these drugs are preliminary, and much remains to be learned about the side effects of the drugs. As a media advisory statement released by the American Heart Association (1997) notes, researchers know little about the prevalence of valvular damage, which patients are at high risk, or whether the damage is reversible when the drugs are discontinued. Future reports will undoubtedly shed more light on these and other questions about the safety of fenfluramine and dexfenfluramine.

Although more definitive recommendations should emerge as more data become available, patients who have taken dexfenfluramine or fenfluramine are advised to talk with their physician and undergo a physical examination. Echocardiography may be helpful for patients who have signs or symptoms of valvular damage or pulmonary hypertension or show evidence of these disorders on clinical evaluation. Signs or symptoms of these disorders can include heart murmur, shortness of breath, tightness in the chest, and swelling in the lower extremities. Patients with valve damage are advised to take an antibiotic before dental or surgical procedures that introduce bacteria into the bloodstream.

Events surrounding the release and withdrawal of dexfenfluramine and fenfluramine underscore the fact that there is no magic cure for obesity. Risks of taking any antiobesity drug must be weighed against the risks of remaining obese. As stated throughout this course, permanent dietary, lifestyle, and exercise changes remain the cornerstones of all obesity management strategies.

SURGERY

Surgical intervention for obesity is considered appropriate only for individuals with

1. Morbid obesity (actual weight exceeding desirable weight by 100 pounds or 100 percent or more)

2. Obesity-related medical problems

3. In whom other weight loss measure have repeatedly failed (Skelton, 1992)

Before 1980, jejunoileal bypass surgery, where a portion of the small intestine was removed, was the most common form of surgery for obesity. Since 1980 this type of surgery has been largely replaced by other types of surgeries because of the numerous complications and high mortality rate (Perri, 1992).

Today two main types of surgeries are used to treat morbid obesity (Kral, 1995)

•   Gastric restriction

•   Combined gastric restriction and malabsorption

With gastric restriction, the size and capacity of the stomach are limited. The stomach pouch is reduced to a 15 ml pouch. Gastric restriction can be accomplished by using a vertical band of staples with a banded outlet *(Figure 9.1)* or by circumgastric banding. With circumgastric banding, an inflatable band connected to a subcutaneous reservoir limits the size of the stomach. Circumgastric banding is a less invasive procedure and may be used in patients considered poor risks for other types of surgeries. Circumgastric banding can now be performed by laparoscope, further reducing invasiveness and risk.

Limitations of gastric restriction are that some higher-calorie soft foods such as cookies, chocolate, or potato chips can pass through the pouch quickly.

FIGURE 9.1
Vertical stapled gastroplasty with a banded outlet from the 15-milliliter pouch

15 ml

9 mm

Source: Kral, J. G. (1995). Surgical interventions for obesity. In K. D. Brownell, & C. G. Fairburn, (Eds.). *Eating disorders and obesity,* (pp. 510–515). New York: The Guilford Press.

FIGURE 9.2
Gastric bypass excluding most of the stomach, the duodenum, and a 40 to 50 centimeter segment of proximal jejunum.

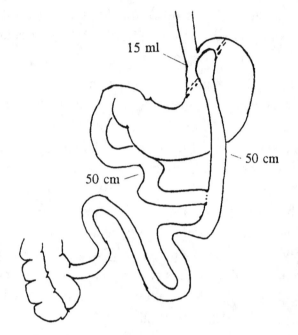

15 ml

50 cm

50 cm

Source: Kral, J. G. (1995). Surgical interventions for obesity. In K. D. Brownell, & C. G. Fairburn, (Eds.). *Eating disorders and obesity,* (pp. 510–515). New York: The Guilford Press.

Also, repeated overdistending can stretch the pouch. Sometimes a second surgery is necessary.

Finally, some patients may be unwilling to modify their eating behavior.

The second type of gastric surgery, combined gastric restriction and malabsorption, is illustrated in *Figure 9.2*. This type of surgery combines a small stomach pouch with the bypass of 90 percent of the stomach, the duodenum, and a limb of jejunum of varying length (Kral, 1995). When high-calorie foods are dumped into the limb of the small intestine, a feeling of satiety or even discomfort may result, helping to curb appetite. Gastric restriction combined with malabsorption is a more aggressive approach than gastric restriction alone. It also results in more postsurgical complications, but may yield greater weight losses. Kral (1995) recommends a stepped-care approach to surgical

intervention for obesity, with laparoscopic banding offered as a first step followed by more aggressive degrees of gastric malabsorption procedures and gastric restriction if laparoscopic banding fails.

Kral (1995) notes that mortality rate for these types of surgeries is less than 0.5 percent if performed by competent physicians, which is less than the mortality rate for morbid obesity left untreated. As with other types of aggressive obesity interventions, surgery for obesity should be used in the context of a comprehensive dietary and physical activity program. Use of antiobesity drugs may also help postsurgical patients who have reached a weight-loss plateau during follow-up.

The next chapter describes nutritional interventions for individuals with eating disorders.

EXAM QUESTIONS

CHAPTER 9
Questions 61–66

61. Very low-calorie diets usually provide what number of calories daily?

    a. less than 500

    b. 500 to 800

    c. 800 to 1,000

    d. 1,200 or more

62. A low-dose multivitamin and mineral supplement would probably be advisable on a diet providing which number of calories daily?

    a. 1,500

    b. 1,800

    c. 1,000

    d. 2,100

63. The lower the calorie content of the diet, the

    a. lower the carbohydrate content should be

    b. lower the protein content should be

    c. lower the fat content should be

    d. the higher the fat content should be

64. The anti-obesity drugs fenfluramine and dexfenfluramine were voluntarily withdrawn from the market by their manufacturers because of concerns of increased risk of which of the following?

    a. Colon cancer

    b. Depression

    c. Heart valve damage

    d. Ulcers

65. Patients who discontinued taking fenfluramine or dexfenfluramine should

    a. talk with their doctor and undergo a physical exam

    b. be alert for symptoms of depression

    c. undergo a complete GI series

    d. increase dietary fiber content of the diet

66. What surgical procedure refers to limiting the size and capacity of the stomach by either a vertical band of staples or by circumgastric banding?

    a. gastric malabsorption

    b. gastric restriction

    c. gastric bypass

    d. jejunoileal bypass

CHAPTER 10

INTERVENTION: NUTRITIONAL MANAGEMENT OF EATING DISORDERS

CHAPTER OBJECTIVE

After reading this chapter, you will be able to recognize key components of nutritional management of patients with anorexia nervosa or bulimia nervosa.

LEARNING OBJECTIVES

After studying this chapter, you will be able to

1. Specify the nurse's role as part of a multidisciplinary health care team in nutritional management of patients with eating disorders.

2. Identify nutritional management goals for patients with anorexia nervosa or bulimia nervosa.

3. Select appropriate energy intakes and meal patterns for nutritional rehabilitation of patients with eating disorders.

4. Recognize elements of education and counseling that promote long-term recovery from an eating disorder.

INTRODUCTION

As discussed in chapter six, nutritional therapy and repletion is central to all methods of treating patients with eating disorders. Psychological approaches such as cognitive behavioral therapy, behavioral therapy, psychoeducation, psychotherapy, or family therapy will do little good if the patient is so malnourished or controlled by erratic eating behavior that he or she has no energy left to concentrate on therapy. Nutrition intervention for patients with eating disorders should therefore be started early in therapy and continue simultaneously with psychological therapy.

This chapter will review the nurse's role in nutrition intervention for eating disorders in the context of a multidisciplinary team setting. Goals of nutritional management will be discussed, and guidelines will be given for selecting appropriate energy and nutritional contents of diets for patients with anorexia nervosa or bulimia nervosa. Components of education, recovery, and maintenance will also be described.

A MULTIDISCIPLINARY TEAM APPROACH

Because many complex factors interact to cause and maintain an eating disorder, the ideal setting for management of eating disorders is multidisciplinary in nature. Each team member contributes a different area of expertise, and all work together to help the patient achieve common goals. Whether management of eating disorders is done on an inpatient or outpatient bases, there should be as much continuity of care as possible, with members of the team providing continued counseling and follow-up over the long-term if possible.

The multidisciplinary team is usually composed of physicians, psychiatrists, psychologists, nurses, social workers, occupational therapists, and dietitians. The psychologist or the psychiatric clinical nurse specialist provide psychological assessment, planning, therapy, and evaluation. The two main responsibilities of the physician are to assess the medical condition of the patient and to discuss treatment options with other team members. The occupational therapist works with other team members to help patients achieve psychological, social, and physical competence.

Dietitians are trained in nutritional assessment and instruction, but may have varying degrees of experience working with eating disordered patients. Dietitians specially trained in management of eating disorders should be available to provide ongoing education and counseling. Usually, the dietitian devises the nutritional care plan, but all members of the management team are responsible for carrying the plan out.

THE NURSE'S ROLE

Nurses usually have more direct patient contact than any other member of the management team and can provide continual feedback and encouragement as the patient works to develop a realistic body image, change irrational attitudes toward food, reduce anxiety, and correct misperceptions (Stephenson and colleagues, 1988). Inpatient nurses are responsible for 24-hour care of the patient. Outpatient nurses provide frequent contact and symptom monitoring. Nurses are also actively involved in the management team and provide other team members with information and feedback to help devise effective management plans.

Inpatient Nursing

Nurses on an inpatient eating disorders facility closely supervise patients and monitor symptoms such as eating and purging behavior. They also provide therapeutic intervention in the form of disrupting the bingeing, purging, or avoidance cycles the patient has become obsessed with. Some of the responsibilities of nurses in inpatient eating disorder units include (Stephenson and colleagues, 1988)

- Measuring body weight daily in a consistent manner (usually in the morning, after voiding, and in a hospital gown). Nurses must assess whether the patient manipulates weight by water loading, refusing to void, or using concealed objects as weights. If weight accuracy is questionable, the nurse can take a second weight measurement an hour or two later.

- Supervising patients at meals to monitor calorie intake and encourage positive eating behavior and attitudes.

- Observing patients after meals to reduce the opportunity to vomit.

- Providing bathroom supervision to monitor purging behavior such as vomiting or use of laxatives.

In one-to-one daily contact, nurses can assist and support patients as they struggle to change their perceptions about food and body weight, allow patients to express their feelings, mirror these feelings back as the patient begins to recognize them, and assist the patient in setting goals and gaining independence.

Outpatient Nursing

The outpatient nurse at an eating disorders facility assists in initial screening, assessment, and development of a management plan. Outpatient nurses often coordinate treatment among members of the multidisciplinary team. Nurses can provide long-term counseling and support as they monitor symptoms and help the patient adopt new attitudes about eating and body weight. Some of the responsibilities of nurses in an outpatient eating disorder facility include (Stephenson and colleagues, 1988)

- Monitor medical status and symptoms such as weight, electrolytes, blood pressure, pulse, menstrual status, and bingeing and purging behavior.

- Teach the patient self-monitoring, such as keeping food records and documenting feelings.

- Encourage self-rewarding, such as using a pleasurable activity in place of bingeing.

- Help the patient with time management and restructuring.

- Help the patient with problem solving and practicing alternative responses.

- Teach appropriate assertive responses and practice these responses with the patient.

- Challenge faulty cognitive thoughts and feelings that help maintain the eating disorder.

- Provide education, suggestion, and emotional support.

ESTABLISHING A TRUST RELATIONSHIP

Effective counseling of patients with eating disorders depends on the formation of a trust relationship between therapist and patient. Nurses working with patients with eating disorders should strive to be supportive, nonjudgmental, empathetic, and respectful. Once the nurse has gained the trust of the patient, goals and means to achieve them can be mutually set, destructive behaviors can be self-reported—providing a learning opportunity for the patient—and compliance with the management plan increased.

Initially, nurses act as guardians of the patient's health (Irwin, 1993). They provide factual medical and nutritional information and clearly describe treatment goals and objectives. Patients may at first view nurses as their jailers, disrupting the patient's

sense of control and forcing them to face negative emotions that may have been channeled into the eating disorder.

As the patient begins to feel better and as the trust relationship is established, the nurse assumes the role of counselor and advocate. Nurses encourage patients to self-report behavior that perpetuates the eating disorder and use these incidents to educate patients and encourage appropriate responses. When the trust relationship is established, the patient can actively participate in goal setting and developing new attitudes and behaviors, increasing compliance with the management plan.

GOALS OF NUTRITIONAL MANAGEMENT

The ultimate goal or nutrition therapy is to have a patient take responsibility for his or her own eating and to eat normally and sensibly. Although the nurse must be a sympathetic advocate and involve the patient in his or her care, there is no room for compromise in setting the initial goals of nutrition therapy. These are

- To attain and maintain normal nutritional status in adults and also normal growth in adolescents

- To develop normal eating behavior

- To promote a normal attitude toward food

- To promote normal responses to hunger and satiety cues (Beaumont and Touyz, 1995)

Goals of nutrition therapy should be clearly explained to the patient and family members at the outset of therapy. These goals apply whether the patient is being treated on an inpatient or outpatient basis.

To achieve these goals, nurses and other health professionals must work on many levels of care simultaneously. At the outset of treatment, a specific meal plan that provides patients with structure and helps them regain control over their eating is used. Small amounts of high-calorie foods or foods that patients fear or avoid are gradually introduced, desensitizing patients. Thoughts, attitudes, and behaviors relating to body image, relationships, and food are addressed with psychological therapy and education. As therapy progresses, underlying issues that helped create the eating disorder are dealt with.

NUTRITIONAL MANAGEMENT OF PATIENTS WITH ANOREXIA NERVOSA

Nutritional rehabilitation of patients with anorexia nervosa can be done on an inpatient or outpatient basis. Patients who have serious medical complications (such as anemia, edema, cachexia, or acute dilation of the stomach), patients with very low body weights, patients with severe behavioral disturbances, patients who need to be separated from the family or partner, and patients who fail to respond to outpatient therapy are candidates for hospitalization (Fichter, 1995).

Because of increasing monetary pressures and other factors, more and more patients with anorexia nervosa are being treated on an outpatient basis. Many day-patient centers are now evolving for the management of patients with eating disorders.

The primary nutritional problem of patients with anorexia nervosa is inadequate calorie intake, and the primary goal is to increase energy intake to restore normal body weight. Although some patients have varying degrees of other nutritional deficiencies, restoring adequate calorie intake usually reverses these deficiencies. Very few patients require nutritional supplementation, and since the ultimate goal of therapy is to eat normally and sensibly, prescribing a modified diet only reinforces the patient's belief that he or she cannot eat nor-

mally (Beaumont and Touyz, 1995).

Target body weights are those maintained by eating a normal, healthy diet without restriction and by exercising moderately and sensibly on a regular basis. For adults, healthy target weights should be between 20 and 25 BMI units. For children and younger adolescents, growth charts provide guidance on healthy body weights. Since growth may already be stunted, growth potential must be used as a guide.

A meal plan intended to promote a weight gain of two to four pounds weekly is designed based on a patient's individual food history. The initial calorie level is low, around 1,200 to 1,500 calories daily, and is increased slowly as the patient becomes accustomed to eating again. Eventually an intake of as high as 3,500 calories daily may be needed, occasionally requiring use of a concentrated, high-calorie product.

Patients should be encouraged to eat in a group setting—such as eating with other patients and staff on an inpatient basis—to provide role models and an opportunity to socialize. Nurses should try to avoid confrontation during mealtimes and provide encouragement and counseling in a positive manner.

NUTRITIONAL MANAGEMENT OF PATIENTS WITH BULIMIA NERVOSA

The primary nutritional problem in patients with bulimia nervosa is a chaotic pattern of eating where periods of overly restrained eating alternate with periods of bingeing. Since most individuals with bulimia nervosa are close to normal weight, these individuals do not need to gain weight. Rather, nutritional therapy for patients with bulimia nervosa should focus on helping patients regain control over their eating, relearn how to eat normally in response to hunger and satiety cues, avoid restrictive dieting practices, and accept a body weight that may be higher than they would like.

Initially a specific meal plan may provide needed structure and help the patient regain control over his or her eating. Meal plans can provide six small meals daily to help reduce binge eating. Patients are instructed to resume this meal plan even after episodes of bingeing without compensating for calories taken in the binge episode. Nurses can educate patients about the futility and risks of purging behaviors, which are also monitored and recorded.

Eventually, the focus should shift to normal, relaxed eating in response to hunger and satiety cues and avoidance of restrained eating and dieting. Nurses should encourage patients to accept their normal body weight as that which occurs with normal eating and regular, sensible exercise even though that weight may be considerably higher than their current weight.

Individuals with bulimia nervosa often avoid or fear certain foods—often the high-calorie foods that they binge on. Small amounts of these foods should be introduced gradually, helping the patient to realize that a normal diet can also include moderate amounts of high-calorie foods.

Most counseling for bulimia nervosa is done on an outpatient basis. Therapy should be weekly or biweekly at first and then gradually less frequently as patients take increasing responsibility and regain control over their eating. If the patient experiences relapse, he or she should immediately return to a structured meal plan and renew therapist contact.

DEVELOPING A MEAL PLAN

The steps in calculating a meal plan for patients with eating disorders are essentially the same as those used in calculating a meal plan for weight loss (see chapter eight on conservative management of obesity). First, energy needs are determined. For individuals with bulimia nervosa, a general guideline of 10 to 12 calories per pound of actual body weight for sedentary individuals, 13 to 15 calories per pound for moderately active individuals, and 16 to 20 calories per pound for very active individuals can be used.

However, individuals with bulimia nervosa may be slightly under normal weight, so a slightly higher figure may be more appropriate. An alternative approach is to set a calorie level that satisfies the patient's appetite. Setting a calorie level below calorie requirements should be avoided, since this reinforces the patient's fear of becoming fat and imposes dietary restrictions, which in turn promote binge behaviors.

For individuals with anorexia nervosa, a 1,200- to 1,500-calorie diet is initially prescribed, since energy intake has been suboptimal for extended periods of time and higher energy intakes initially might cause discomfort. Food can be divided into six smaller meals to decrease discomfort. Energy intake is then gradually increased in 300-calorie increments at a time until the patient reaches a healthy body weight. Calorie intake is not increased until the patient manages to complete each meal and snack. Some patients, especially those who have abused laxatives, may require a stool softener or a diet generous in dietary fiber to promote regularity.

After energy level is determined, calories are distributed into grams of proteins, carbohydrates, and fats using the figures of 4 calories per gram for carbohydrates and proteins and 9 calories per gram for fats. At normal calorie levels, the recommended distribution of nutrients for individuals with eating disorders is the same as for the general public

- Less than 30 percent of calories as fat

- About 50 to 55 percent of calories as carbohydrates

- About 15 percent of calories as proteins (with a minimum of 44 grams high-quality proteins for women and about 56 grams for men

- 20 to 30 grams dietary fiber

- Less than 200 milligrams of cholesterol daily

However, for patients initiating therapy on 1,200- to 1,500-calorie diets, the percentage of proteins may be slightly greater than 15 to obtain adequate high-quality protein intake. Further, for patients on very high-calorie intakes—for example, 3,500 calories daily—the percentage of calories from fat may be slightly higher than 30 since the patients may have difficulty consuming such a large volume of food.

Grams of proteins, carbohydrates, and fats are then translated into number of servings from the food exchange lists (see *Tables 8.2 and 8.3*), and servings from the exchange lists are divided into meals and snacks.

As the patient gains weight or stabilizes his or her eating pattern, small amounts of problem foods are incorporated into the meal plan. After a healthy body weight has been reestablished and after the patient assumes responsibility for normal, healthy eating, spontaneous eating based on hunger and satiety cues resumes. The meal plan then serves as a structured backup in times of relapse.

Sample Initial Meal Plan for a Patient with Anorexia Nervosa

The 1,500-calorie meal plan shown below might be used for the first 7 to 10 days of nutritional rehabilitation of a patient with anorexia nervosa. Slightly lower initial calorie levels might be appropriate for some patients, while higher intakes might be appropriate for others. After the patient adapts to the initial calorie level, calories are gradually increased as tolerated by the patient until a healthy body weight is reached.

1,500-Calorie Meal Plan

7 starch exchanges

5 lean or medium-fat meat exchanges

4 vegetable exchanges

3 fruit exchanges

3 skim or low-fat milk exchanges

3 fat exchanges

Breakfast

1 starch exchange	1 slice whole wheat toast
1 fat exchange	1 teaspoon margarine
1 lean meat exchange	1 boiled egg
1 milk exchange	1 cup skim milk
1 fruit exchange	1/2 grapefruit

Morning Snack

1 starch exchange	8 animal crackers

Lunch

2 starch exchanges	2 slices pumpernickel bread
1 lean meat exchange	1 ounce sliced chicken breast
1 fat exchange	1 teaspoon mayonnaise
1 vegetable exchange	1/2 cup cooked carrots
1 fruit exchange	1/2 cup canned pineapple
1 milk exchange	1 cup skim milk

Afternoon Snack

1 vegetable exchange	1/2 cup tomato juice
1 starch exchange	3/4 ounce Matzoh

Supper

2 starch exchanges	1 cup rice
3 lean meat exchanges	3 ounces thinly-sliced beefround
2 vegetable exchanges	1 cup steamed pea pods
1 fat	1 teaspoon oil to cook beef, pea pods in

Evening Snack

1 milk exchange	nonfat yogurt
1 fruit exchange	1 small banana

Sample Meal Plan for a Patient with Bulimia Nervosa

The following 2,000-calorie meal plan might be appropriate for an adult woman with bulimia nervosa weighing 150 pounds and measuring 5'8" tall.

Sample 2,000-Calorie Meal Plan

9 starch exchanges

6 lean or medium-fat meat exchanges

5 vegetable exchanges

4 fruit exchanges

3 skim or low-fat milk exchanges

5 fat exchanges

Breakfast

2 starch exchanges	1 whole bagel
1 fat exchange	1 tablespoon cream cheese
1 fruit exchange	1¼ cups whole fresh strawberries
1 milk exchange	1 cup skim milk

Morning Snack

1 starch exchange	2 small fat-free cookies
1 fruit exchange	1/2 cup orange juice

Lunch

1 starch exchange	24 oyster crackers
1 meat and 1 starch exchange	1/2 cup cooked lentils in soup
2 vegetable exchanges	1/2 cup cooked vegetables in soup
1 fat	1 teaspoon margarine in soup
1 fruit	3/4 cup blueberries

Afternoon Snack

1 starch and 1 fat exchange	1 brownie, 2" square
1 milk exchange	1 cup skim milk

Supper

2 starch exchanges	1 small baked potato and 1 small dinner roll
1 fat exchange	1 teaspoon margarine
5 medium-fat meat exchanges	5-ounce prime rib
2 vegetable exchanges	1 cup cooked broccoli
1 fruit exchange	1/2 cup canned peaches packed in own juice

Evening Snack

1 starch exchange	3 cups low-fat microwave popcorn
1 vegetable exchange	1 cup raw carrot sticks

MONITORING THE MEAL PLAN

When developing a meal plan, calorie levels are only estimated and usually need adjusting. If a patient experiences significant hunger, calorie levels should be increased to prevent bingeing. If a patient loses weight and is eating all the food in the current meal plan without purging, calorie levels should be increased. Weekly or biweekly weighing is necessary as the meal plan is adjusted.

The patient can assist the initial monitoring process by keeping a daily food diary, such as the one shown in *Figure 8.1*. In addition to recording level of hunger, physical position, where, when, what, and how much was eaten, patients can also note frequency of binge/purge episodes, weight fluctuations, perceived level of control when the food was eaten, and any emotions they were feeling either before or after eating. Nurses and dietitians can review the daily food record at each visit and use it as an instructional tool to promote and reinforce positive changes in eating behaviors and attitudes. Some patients, however, become obsessed with record keeping. For these patients, a less structured form of self monitoring may be helpful.

EDUCATION AND COUNSELING

Although patients with eating disorders may appear highly knowledgeable about nutritional matters and can quote endless calorie values for various foods, nurses and other health professionals should not assume that these patients are well-informed about nutrition and healthy eating. Individuals with eating disorders are often selective in what information they believe and obtain their information from questionable sources, such as popular magazines. They also can distort nutritional information to justify their particular eating behaviors.

Nutritional counseling and education is a critical component for patients with eating disorders to correct misinformation and provide accurate knowledge of nutritional and caloric requirements. Families should also be included in this effort, since their nutritional knowledge may also be limited and the patient may misrepresent information given. Topics to be included in educational sessions include (Beaumont and Touyz, 1995)

- The energy equation and balance of energy intake, expenditure, and body weight

- Nutrient content of foods

- Dangers of dieting and purging behaviors

- Changing dietary requirements as weight is regained

- Nutritional requirements for good health and weight maintenance

RECOVERY AND MAINTENANCE

Once a nutritional rehabilitation and eating stabilization are achieved, continued therapist contact and monitoring are needed to assure patients do not revert back to old patterns of eating and behavior. The average recovery time for patients with eating disorders is five or more years, so nurses and therapists should expect periods of relapse and maintain continued, although less frequent, contact with patients. Patients should be encouraged to return to a structured meal pattern and return to therapy immediately when they experience major episodes of relapse.

The maintenance period is often an unsettling time for patients with eating disorders, since they lack the security of a highly structured meal plan. During this maintenance period, patients practice new attitudes and behaviors in a variety of settings, such as eating at home or eating out at a restaurant. Patients plan and rehearse responses ahead of time under the guidance of the health care team. Relapses are inevitable and are viewed as learning opportunities.

The next chapter reviews management of obesity and eating disorders in special populations.

EXAM QUESTIONS

CHAPTER 10
Questions 67–74

67. Which health professional often has more direct contact with patients with eating disorders than any other member of the treatment team?

a. nurse

b. dietitian

c. physician

d. psychologist

68. Effective counseling of patients with eating disorders depends on

a. support of family members or spouses

b. formation of a trust relationship between therapist and patient

c. accurate monitoring of eating and purging behaviors

d. firm control of dietary intake

69. An initial goal of nutrition therapy for a patient with an eating disorder is to

a. teach life-long monitoring of all foods and beverages consumed

b. help the patient learn to eat at scheduled times

c. attain and maintain normal nutritional status

d. increase body weight by 5 percent

70. The primary nutritional problem for patients with anorexia nervosa is inadequate intake of

a. protein

b. calories

c. iron

d. calcium

71. Which of the following regarding nutritional repletion of patients with anorexia nervosa is true?

a. Initial calorie intake should be set at 2,500 to 3,000 calories daily to regain weight as rapidly as possible.

b. Calorie intakes are not adjusted until the psychological factors causing the eating disorder have been addressed.

c. Initial calorie intakes are set at 500 to 600 calories daily and are increased at 500-calorie increments weekly.

d. Initial calorie intakes are set at around 1,200 to 1,500 calories daily and are increased gradually as the patient becomes accustomed to eating again.

72. The primary nutritional problem in patients with bulimia nervosa is

    a. a chaotic pattern of eating where periods of overly restrained eating alternate with periods of bingeing

    b. inadequate calorie intake

    c. excessive calorie intake

    d. inadequate intake of key vitamins and minerals

73. Which of the following is true regarding patients with eating disorders?

    a. They are usually very knowledgeable about nutrition.

    b. They usually know very little about nutrition.

    c. They are not interested in nutrition.

    d. They may appear knowledgeable about nutrition but may have selective knowledge or nutrition misinformation.

74. The average recovery time for patients with eating disorders is

    a. 6 months

    b. 1 year

    c. 3 years

    d. 5 or more years

CHAPTER 11

INTERVENTION: OBESITY AND EATING DISORDERS IN SPECIAL POPULATIONS

CHAPTER OBJECTIVE

After reading this chapter, you will be able to recognize unique dietary management considerations for special groups of patients with obesity or eating disorders.

LEARNING OBJECTIVES

After studying this chapter, you will be able to

1. Recognize unique aspects of management of obesity in children, elderly patients, and patients with non-insulin-dependent diabetes, atherosclerosis, high blood pressure, or cancer.

2. Recognize unique aspects of management of eating disorders in males, preadolescent, athletes, the elderly, and patients who have been sexually abused or who have non-insulin-dependent diabetes.

INTRODUCTION

Certain subgroups of patients have special nutritional needs which make their medical management unique from the general population. This chapter will review dietary aspects of obesity management and prevention for individuals with non-insulin-dependent (type II) diabetes, atherosclerosis, high blood pressure, or cancer. Obesity in the elderly and young will be discussed. This chapter will also discuss management of eating disorders in subgroups of patients, including males, younger children, athletes, the elderly, and patients with non-insulin-dependent diabetes.

MANAGEMENT OF OBESITY IN SPECIAL POPULATIONS

Non-Insulin-Dependent Diabetes

Non-insulin-dependent, or type II, diabetes is one of the leading causes of death in the United States. Type II diabetes usually develops later in life and resists treatment.

Obesity is one of the main risk factors for the development of type II diabetes. About 80 percent of individuals with type II diabetes are obese. Obesity aggravates diabetes by raising blood sugar levels and increasing insulin resistance. Weight loss usually decreases the need for medication or insulin in type II diabetes and may even reverse the disease.

Weight loss is a primary goal for obese individuals with type II diabetes, along with goals of maintaining normal blood glucose, blood lipid, and blood pressure levels (American Diabetes Association, 1996). Meal plans for obese individuals with type II diabetes should be designed to help them reach and maintain reasonable weight goals over the long-term. Although achieving an ideal body weight would be desirable, this goal is not practical for many individuals. Even modest weight losses of 10 to 20 pounds can produce significant improvements in individuals with type II diabetes.

Based on nutrition recommendations of the American Diabetes Association (1996), recommended diets for most patients with type II diabetes are similar to recommended diets for the general population and should provide

- 10 to 20 percent of daily calories from protein

- Less than 30 percent of total calories from fat

- Less than 10 percent of total calories from saturated fat

- 20 to 35 grams of dietary fiber from foods

- Modest decrease in calories (250 to 500 calories) compared to calorie intake on usual diet, which should be complemented by a modest increase in calories burned from physical activity

- No restriction in sugar intake

For most of this century, health experts have advised individuals with diabetes to restrict their intake of simple sugars. The American Diabetes Association, however, has concluded that little scientific evidence exists to support this conclusion.

Although these are general guidelines, diets must be individualized for each patient based on lifestyle, existing habits, and diabetes management goals. Individuals with type II diabetes who also have high blood cholesterol levels, for example, may need to follow a more fat-restricted diet. Individuals with high blood pressure may need to restrict sodium intake.

Atherosclerosis

Fear of the number-one killer in the United States, heart disease, has been a powerful motivator for many Americans to modify their diets. Obesity, particularly abdominal obesity, increases the risk of atherosclerotic cardiovascular disease both independently and through its effects on blood pressure,

blood lipids, and blood glucose levels (Bierman, 1992).

High blood cholesterol levels, especially high levels of low-density lipoprotein (LDL) cholesterol, are associated with greater risk of coronary heart disease (CHD). Another type of lipoprotein, high-density lipoprotein (HDL) cholesterol, helps protect against CHD. The risk for CHD rises progressively with blood cholesterol levels above 200 mg/dl. Risk sharply rises with cholesterol levels above 220 mg/dl.

According to guidelines of the National Cholesterol Education Program of the National Institutes of Health (1993), a desirable blood cholesterol level for all adults is below 200 mg/dl. A level between 200 and 239 mg/dl is considered borderline-high, and a level of 240 mg/dl or greater is considered high.

All individuals should be given preventative diet information to reduce risk of heart disease. Obese individuals at risk for heart disease need to lose weight and lower total fat, saturated fat, and cholesterol content of their diet. These diet goals should also be actively pursued in individuals who have already experienced a heart attack (Rossouw, 1990).

For individuals with borderline-high or high blood cholesterol levels, diet therapy and exercise is the first line of treatment, followed by a combination of diet and drug therapy if response to diet therapy is inadequate after six months (or sooner if lipids are severely-elevated). *Table 11.1* lists blood total and LDL cholesterol level goals of diet therapy for high blood cholesterol levels.

Diet therapy can be implemented in a two-step fashion, as shown in *Table 11.2*. The Step-One Diet advocated in the National Cholesterol Education Program (1993) contains 30 percent or less of calories from fat, 8 to 10 percent of calories from saturated fat, and less than 300 mg of dietary cholesterol daily. The Step-Two Diet goes a little

---

TABLE 11.1 Blood Total and LDL Cholesterol Level Goals of Nutrition Therapy

	Initiation Level	Goal of Therapy	Monitoring Goal
	LDL-cholesterol		*Total cholesterol*
Without CHD and with fewer than 2 risk factors	≥160 mg/dL	<160 mg/dL	<240 mg/dL
Without CHD and with 2 or more risk factors	≤130 mg/dL	<130 mg/dL	<200 mg/dL
With CHD	>100 mg/dL	≤100 mg/dL	≤160 mg/dL

Source: National Institutes of Health. (1993). *The fifth report of the Joint National Committee on Detection, Evaluation, and Treatment of High Blood Pressure.* Washington, D.C.: U.S. Government Printing Office. NIH Publication No. 93–1088.

---

further by limiting saturated fat intake to seven percent of calories and limiting dietary cholesterol to 200 milligrams daily. The Step-Two Diet is used when response to the Step-One Diet is inadequate.

Most of the changes in the Step-One Diet can be made without drastically altering dietary patterns. The Step-Two Diet will require more careful attention to food selection. Recommended diet modifications for the Step-One and Step-Two Diets are shown in *Table 11.3*. These diets for lowering serum lipid levels are very similar to recommendations of the American Heart Association. *Table 11.4* gives minimum daily intake of fat and saturated fatty acids to achieve Step-One or Step-Two Diets. In addition, *Table 11.5* lists the fat, saturated fat, and cholesterol values in different types of meat, poultry, and fish to help in meal planning of Step-One and Step-Two diets.

Many researchers believe that soluble dietary fiber—the type found in oat products, dried beans and peas, and many fruits and vegetables—helps lower blood cholesterol (Anderson and Gustafson, 1988). Since these foods are also very low in fat and contain no cholesterol, patients can be encouraged to include moderate amounts of these foods in a cholesterol-lowering diet.

The omega-3 fatty acids found in oily fish like salmon, mackerel, haddock and other cold water fish may help protect against heart disease. In populations who consume large quantities of such fish, like the Greenland Eskimos, heart disease is virtually nonexistent. Although omega-3 fatty acid supplements are not recommended, patients should be encouraged to eat fish often. Fish (providing it is baked or poached rather than fried) is still fairly low in fat and calories compared to many other protein foods.

TABLE 11.2 Diet Therapy for High Blood Cholesterol Levels

NUTRIENT*		RECOMMENDED INTAKE	
	Step-I Diet		**Step-II Diet**
Total Fat		30% or less of	
Saturated Fatty Acids	8-10% of total calories	total calories	Less than 7% of total calories
Polyunsaturated Fatty Acids		Up to 10% of total calories	
Monounsaturated Fatty Acids		Up to 15% of total calories	
Carbohydrates		55% or more of total calories	
Protein		Approximately 15% of total calories	
Cholesterol	Less than 300 mg/day		Less than 200 mg/day
Total Calories		To achieve and maintain desirable weight	

* *Calories from alcohol not included.*

Source: National Institutes of Health. (1993). *The fifth report of the Joint National Committee on Detection, Evaluation, and Treatment of High Blood Pressure.* Washington, D.C.: U.S. Government Printing Office. NIH Publication No. 93–1088.

TABLE 11.3 Recommended Dietary Changes for Step-I and Step-II Diets*

Food Group	Choose	Decrease
Lean Meat, Poultry, and Fish ≤5-6 oz. per day	Beef, pork, lamb—lean cuts well trimmed before cooking	Beef, pork, lamb—regular ground beef, fatty cuts, spare ribs, organ meats
	Poultry without skin	Poultry with skin, fried chicken
	Fish, shellfish	Fried fish, fried shellfish
	Processed meat—prepared from lean meat, e.g., lean ham, lean frankfurters, lean meat with soy protein or carrageenan	Regular luncheon meat, e.g., bologna, salami, sausage, frankfurters
Eggs ≤4 yolks per week, Step I ≤2 yolks per week, Step II	Egg whites (two whites can be substituted for one whole egg in recipes), cholesterol-free egg substitute	Egg yolks (if more than four per week on Step I or if more than two per week on Step II); includes eggs used in cooking and baking
Low-Fat Dairy Products 2-3 servings per day	Milk—skim, 1/2%, or 1% fat (fluid, powdered, evaporated), buttermilk	Whole milk (fluid, evaporated, condensed), 2% fat milk (lowfat milk), imitation milk
	Yogurt—nonfat or low-fat yogurt or yogurt beverages	Whole milk yogurt, whole milk yogurt beverages
	Cheese—low-fat natural or processed cheese	Regular cheeses (American, blue, Brie, cheddar, Colby, Edam, Monterey Jack, whole-milk mozzarella, Parmesan, Swiss), cream cheese, Neufchatel cheese
	Low-fat or nonfat varieties, e.g.: cottage cheese—low-fat, nonfat, or dry curd (0 to 2% fat)	Cottage cheese (4% fat)
	Frozen dairy dessert—ice milk, frozen yogurt (low fat or nonfat)	Ice cream
	Low-fat coffee creamer Low-fat or nonfat sour cream	Cream, half & half, whipping cream, nondairy creamer, whipped topping, sour cream

* Careful selection of processed foods is necessary to stay within the sodium <2,400 mg guideline.

Source: National Institutes of Health. (1993). *The fifth report of the Joint National Committee on Detection, Evaluation, and Treatment of High Blood Pressure.* Washington, D.C.: U.S. Government Printing Office. NIH Publication No. 93–1088.

TABLE 11.3 Recommended Dietary Changes for Step-I and Step-II Diets* *(Cont.)*

Food Group	Choose	Decrease
Fats and Oils ≤6–8 teaspoons per day	Unsaturated oils—safflower, sunflower, corn, soybean, cottonseed, canola, olive, peanut	Coconut oil, palm kernel oil, palm oil
	Margarine—made from unsaturated oils listed above, light or diet margarine, especially soft or liquid forms	Butter, lard, shortening, bacon fat, hard margarine
	Salad dressings—made with unsaturated oils listed above, low-fat or fat free	Dressings made with egg yolk, cheese, sour cream, whole milk
	Seeds and nuts—peanut butter, other nut butters	Coconut
	Cocoa powder	Milk chocolate
Breads and Cereals 6 or more servings per day	Breads—whole-grain bread, English muffins, bagels, buns, corn or flour tortilla	Bread in which eggs, fat, and/or butter are a major ingredient; croissants
	Cereals—oat, wheat, corn, multigrain	Most granolas
	Pasta	
	Rice	
	Dry beans and peas	
	Crackers, low-fat—animal-type, graham, soda crackers, breadsticks, melba toast	High-fat crackers
	Homemade baked goods using unsaturated oil, skim or 1% milk, and egg substitute—quick breads, biscuits, cornbread muffins, bran muffins, pancakes, waffles	Commercial baked pastries, muffins, biscuits

Source: National Institutes of Health. (1993). *The fifth report of the Joint National Committee on Detection, Evaluation, and Treatment of High Blood Pressure.* Washington, D.C.: U.S. Government Printing Office. NIH Publication No. 93–1088.

TABLE 11.3 Recommended Dietary Changes for Step-I and Step-II Diets* *(Cont.)*

Food Group	Choose	Decrease
Soups	Reduced- or low-fat and reduced-sodium varieties, e.g., chicken or beef noodle, minestrone, tomato, vegetable, potato, reduced-fat soups made with skim milk	Soup containing whole milk, cream, meat fat, poultry fat, or poultry skin
Vegetables 3–5 servings per day	Fresh, frozen, or canned, without added fat or sauce	Vegetables fried or prepared with butter, cheese, or cream sauce
Fruits 2–4 servings per day	Fruit—fresh, frozen, canned, or dried Fruit juice—fresh, frozen, or canned Beverages—fruit-flavored drinks, lemonade, fruit punch	Fried fruit or fruit served with butter or cream sauce
Sweets and Modified Fat Desserts	Sweets—sugar, syrup, honey, jam, preserves, candy made without fat (candy corn, gumdrops, hard candy), fruit-flavored gelatin	Candy made with milk chocolate, coconut oil, palm kernel oil, palm oil
	Frozen desserts—low-fat and nonfat yogurt, ice milk, sherbet, sorbet, fruit ice, popsicles	Ice cream and frozen treats made with ice cream
	Cookies, cake, pie, pudding—prepared with egg whites, egg substitute, skim milk or 1% milk, and unsaturated oil or margarine; ginger snaps; fig and other fruit bar cookies, fat-free cookies; angel food cake	Commercial baked pies, cakes, doughnuts, high-fat cookies, cream pies

Source: National Institutes of Health. (1993). *The fifth report of the Joint National Committee on Detection, Evaluation, and Treatment of High Blood Pressure.* Washington, D.C.: U.S. Government Printing Office. NIH Publication No. 93–1088.

TABLE 11.4 Minimum Daily Intake of Fat and Saturated Fatty Acids to Achieve Step-I and Step-II Diets[a]

	Total Calorie Level							
	1,600	1,800	2,000	2,200	2,400	2,600	2,800	3,000
Total fat, g[b]	53	60	67	73	80	87	93	100
Saturated fat - Step-I, g[c]	18	20	22	24	27	29	31	33
Saturated fat - Step-II, g[c]	12	14	16	17	19	20	22	23

a   The average daily energy intake for women is about 1,800 calories, for men it is about 2,500 calories.

b   Total fat of both diets = 30 percent of calories (estimated by multiplying calorie level of the diet by 0.3 and dividing the product by 9 calories/gm).

c   The recommended intake of saturated fat on the Step-I Diet should be 8–10 percent of total calories, and less than 7 percent for the Step-II Diet.

Source: National Institutes of Health. (1993). *The fifth report of the Joint National Committee on Detection, Evaluation, and Treatment of High Blood Pressure.* Washington, D.C.: U.S. Government Printing Office. NIH Publication No. 93–1088.

High Blood Pressure

The association of high blood pressure, or hypertension, with obesity has long been recognized (Eliahou, 1992). The Framingham study showed that an excess of body weight only 20 percent over ideal weight was associated with an eight-fold increase in the incidence of high blood pressure later in life. Abdominal obesity is especially associated with high blood pressure.

The goal of treatment for hypertension is to achieve a blood pressure of 140/90 mm Hg or less while controlling other cardiovascular risk factors (National Institutes of Health, 1993). Lifestyle modifications—including weight loss, increased physical activity, and moderation of dietary sodium and alcohol intake—are the first line of treatment for mild high blood pressure and should be tried for three to six months before starting drug therapy. Even when drug therapy is used, lifestyle modifications should continue.

Most importantly, obese individuals with high blood pressure should restrict calories and increased physical activity to lose weight. Even weight losses of as little as 10 pounds will help lower blood pressure (National Institutes of Health, 1993).

Since excessive alcohol intake can raise blood pressure and make drug therapy less effective, alcohol intake should be limited. Alcohol is also a concentrated source of calories that supplies minimal vitamins or minerals. At a maximum, alcoholic beverages should be limited to one ounce of ethanol (two ounces of 100 proof whiskey, eight ounces of wine, or 24 ounces of beer daily).

Many studies show that blood pressure responds to reduced sodium intake, although the response of each individual varies. Blacks, older people, and individuals with high blood pressure seem to be more responsive to sodium intake. The National Institutes of Health (1993) recommends that individuals with mild high blood pressure consume no more than 2.3 grams of sodium daily. Because dietary potassium, calcium and magnesium intakes may be related to blood pressure, adequate intakes of these minerals is recommended.

Salt (sodium chloride) is by far the most plentiful source of sodium in the American Diet. Although sodium is an essential mineral that helps regulate water balance in the body, too much of it serves no purpose and can contribute to increased blood pressure in some individuals sensitive to sodium. We get sodium both in the foods we eat and in the salt that we add to foods. About one-third of the sodium in Americans' diets occurs naturally in the foods we eat. The rest is added via the

TABLE 11.5 Fat, Saturated Fat, Cholesterol, and Iron Content of 3-ounce Portions of Meat, Fish, and Poultry Cooked Without Added Fat

Source	Total Fat g/3 oz	Saturated Fat g/3 oz	Cholesterol mg/3 oz	Iron mg/3 oz
Lean Red Meats				
Beef	4.2	1.4	71	2.5
(rump roast, shank, bottom round, sirloin)				
Lamb	7.8	2.8	78	1.9
(shank roast, sirloin roast, shoulder roast, loin chops, sirloin chops, center leg chop)				
Pork	11.8	4.1	77	1.0
(sirloin cutlet, loin roast, sirloin roast, center roast, butterfly chops, loin chops)				
Veal	4.9	2.0	93	1.0
(blade roast, sirloin chops, shoulder roast, loin chops, rump roast, shank)				
Organ Meats				
Liver				
beef	4.2	1.6	331	5.8
calf	5.9	2.2	477	2.2
chicken	4.6	1.6	537	7.2
Sweetbread	21.3	7.3	250	1.3
Kidney	2.9	0.9	329	6.2
Brains	10.7	2.5	1,747	1.9
Heart	4.8	1.4	164	6.4
Poultry				
Chicken (without skin)				
light (roasted)	3.8	1.1	72	0.9
dark (roasted)	8.3	2.3	79	1.1
Turkey (without skin)				
light (roasted)	2.7	0.9	59	1.1
dark (roasted)	6.1	2.0	72	2.0
Fish				
Haddock	0.8	0.1	63	1.1
Flounder	1.3	0.3	58	0.3
Salmon	7.0	1.7	54	0.3
Tuna, light, canned in water	0.7	0.2	25	1.3
Shellfish				
Crustaceans				
Lobster	0.5	0.1	61	0.3
Crab meat				
Alaskan King	1.3	0.1	45	0.6
Crab Blue Crab	1.5	0.2	85	0.8
Shrimp	0.9	0.2	166	2.6
Mollusks				
Abalone	1.3	0.3	144	5.4
Clams	1.7	0.2	57	23.8
Mussels	3.8	0.7	48	5.7
Oysters	4.2	1.3	93	10.2
Scallops	1.2	0.1	27	2.6
Squid	2.4	0.6	400	1.2

Source: National Institutes of Health. (1993). *The fifth report of the Joint National Committee on Detection, Evaluation, and Treatment of High Blood Pressure.* Washington, D.C.: U.S. Government Printing Office. NIH Publication No. 93–1088.

salt shaker at the table or during cooking.

To limit sodium in the diet

- Decrease use of salt at the table by putting the salt shaker out of sight or disposing of it.

- Do not add salt during cooking. Most recipes calling for salt taste fine without salt, too.

- If foods seem too bland without added salt, sprinkle them with fresh lemon juice. Spices can be substituted for salt also. For example, try adding green pepper, mace, onion, paprika, or parsley to potatoes. Try adding bay leaves, dry mustard, green pepper, marjoram, or fresh mushrooms to beef. Many good salt substitutes are also available.

- Read labels carefully. Many prepared and convenience foods are high in sodium, although more and more companies are making low-sodium prepared foods.

Cancer

Obesity appears to increase risk of developing certain types of cancers. In a study of the American Cancer Society (Garfinkle, 1985), cancer of the endometrium, uterus, cervix, ovary, gallbladder, and breast were increased in obese women. Prostate and colo-rectal cancer were increased in obese men.

The National Cancer Institute gives specific dietary recommendations to help prevent cancer (Butrum and colleagues, 1988). These include

- Reduce fat intake to 30 percent or less of total calories.

- Increase fiber intake to 20 to 30 grams daily.

- Include a variety of vegetables and fruits daily.

- Avoid obesity.

- Consume alcoholic beverages in moderation, if at all.

- Minimize consumption of salt-cured, salt-pickled and smoked foods.

In addition to these recommendations, The National Cancer Institute also encourages Americans to eat more fruits and vegetables. Their campaign promoting this, called "Five a Day for Better Health," recommends eating at least five servings of fruits and vegetables daily. Fruits and vegetables are rich in dietary fiber and also contain compounds called antioxidants, which may help prevent certain cancers.

ELDERLY INDIVIDUALS

Elderly obese patients have special needs due to physiological, socioeconomic, and psychological changes that come with aging. Some older adults may have become obese simply by not reducing food intake as they became more inactive, or by not remaining more active to balance greater food intake. Because there are so many differences among elderly persons and because the past nutrition and physical fitness levels can vary widely, diets for the elderly must be individualized.

As with all medical treatment, the potential benefits of weight loss and weight-management efforts in elderly individuals must be weighed against the perceived costs. If a 78-year old individual needs to lose weight but has no desire to, weight-management efforts may not be appropriate. However, if a 65-year-old individual has obesity-related health problems and is motivated to get his or her weight under control, the nurse and other health professionals can help the patient devise an appropriate weight-management approach. Nurses probably won't see many cases of severely obese elderly individuals, since the severely obese usually die at a younger age.

Many factors should be considered in designing diets for elderly individuals. Body composition changes with age. Weight may decline, but the proportion of body fat increases, almost doubling in men and increasing by 50 percent in women (Andres, 1985).

Many elderly individuals use a variety of over-the-counter or prescription drugs, so possible interactions of foods or alcohol and drugs must be considered. Elderly individuals are also sometimes easy targets for nutritional quackery and may be taking nutritional supplements of questionable value.

Vitamin and mineral absorption decreases with age, so a balanced vitamin and mineral supplement providing 100 percent of the recommended allowances is appropriate for many elderly individuals on balanced calorie-deficit diets.

Calcium is also of special concern to many elderly individuals—especially women—because of the risk or osteoporosis, or brittle bones. The calcium needs of the elderly are at least equivalent to those of younger adults. Some people who have had insufficient calcium intake during adulthood have even higher calcium needs later in life. Other dietary factors also affect the risk of developing osteoporosis

- **Protein intake**—A high-protein intake increases amino acid production and increases loss of calcium, thus countering the effects of increasing calcium intake. If the diet is high in protein, intake of meat and other high protein foods may need to be limited—perhaps to three or four ounces of meat daily.

- **Calcium intake**—The National Institutes of Health conference on osteoporosis recommended a daily calcium intake of 1,000 mg for premenopausal women and postmenopausal women taking estrogen. For postmenopausal women not taking estrogen and all men, a daily intake of 1,500 mg is recommended.

- **Vitamin D**—A reliable source of vitamin D, such as fortified milk, should be ensured since vitamin D is needed to absorb calcium properly.

- **Sodium**—High-sodium intakes increase excretion of calcium in the urine, so sodium intake should be kept in the range of 2 to 4 grams or less of sodium daily.

- **Fat intake**—A high-fat diet decreases the absorption of calcium.

- **Alcohol intake**—Alcohol also decreases absorption of calcium and is toxic to osteoblasts. Alcohol intake should be limited to no more than one alcoholic beverage daily.

- **Caffeine intake**—Patients should limit intake of caffeine to three servings of coffee, tea, or colas daily, since caffeine increases urinary excretion of calcium.

Nurses must also consider other lifestyle factors when designing weight-management programs for elderly individuals. A patient may have difficulty consuming a well-balanced diet if their dentures don't fit right. Likewise, special diets are hard to follow if a person has arthritis and cannot open certain packages of food. Some elderly individuals don't care much about food and eating anymore if they are lonely or have no one to share meals with. Programs such as Meals on Wheels or Congregate Dining can enable elderly persons to enjoy hot, nutritious meals in the company of others.

Children and Adolescents

Just as adult obesity is increasing in prevalence, so is pediatric obesity. About one in four children are overweight, and the numbers are on the rise. Overweight children often, though not always, grow up to be overweight adults. The older the child is at onset of obesity and the more severe the obesity, the greater the chances the child will remain obese as an adult (Dietz, 1992).

Childhood obesity can have severe psychosocial implications. Children who are overweight should not be put on weight loss diets. Many obese children eat the same or fewer calories than normal-weight children (Dietz, 1992). Rather, healthy eating and exercise behaviors should be encouraged to slow the rate of weight gain and allow height to catch up to weight. Severely restricting calories in childhood could interfere with normal growth or promote the development of eating disorders (Johnston, 1985).

With young children, diet counseling should focus on the parents' role as "gatekeepers" of foods brought into the house. If diet assessment reveals the child is eating too many calorically dense foods—such as potato chips, cookies, soft drinks, candy or ice cream—the parents should be encouraged to limit (not necessarily omit) purchase of these foods and try to emphasize healthy meals and snacks.

When counseling older children and adolescents, focusing too much on the parental role may be counterproductive if the child is striving to achieve autonomy. Diet counselors should also be sure that an adolescent who wishes to lose weight really needs to. At any given time, 75 to 95 percent of adolescent girls are dissatisfied with their weight (Obesity Update, 1993).

The nurse should encourage the entire family to adopt healthy eating habits for the benefit of both the patient and other family members. This also avoids singling out the obese child as different or the reason certain foods cannot be kept in the house.

If the child isn't active enough, which is often the case, parents need to encourage activity. This might mean limiting television viewing, allowing adequate time for safe outdoor play, joining a sports team, or planning family activities like nature hikes, swimming, volleyball, sliding or skiing. Although an activity might not be strenuous enough to be considered aerobic, any extra activity helps burn calories.

As with adult obesity, prevention is more effective than treatment. Any child who is above the 75th percentile of weight for height should be monitored closely for development of obesity (The American Dietetic Association, 1989). All children and their parents should be encouraged to adopt healthy eating and exercise behaviors at an early age to help prevent obesity.

MANAGEMENT OF EATING DISORDERS IN SPECIAL POPULATIONS

Males with Eating Disorders

Because most individuals with eating disorders are females, treatment of males with eating disorders has often been neglected, ignored, or dismissed (Andersen, 1995). Males with eating disorders make up about 5 to 15 percent of all individuals with eating disorders, although this number is increasing.

Certain groups of males have increased risk for developing eating disorders. Dieting and eating disorders in males is often related to participation in sports, past obesity, gender identity conflicts, or avoidance of feared medical complications (Anderson, 1995). Male wrestlers have seven to ten times the rate of developing eating disorders compared to all males. Among males with eating disorders, homosexuality is reported in about 21 percent (Andersen, 1995). Males who develop eating disorders are more likely to have been obese in the past than females.

Goals of treatment of males with eating disorders are similar to goals for females. However, males often feel more isolated and apart from therapeutic groups composed mainly of women. Special effort should be made to help male patients with eating disorders realize they are not alone.

Eating Disorders and Athletes

Athletes are at greater risk of developing eating disorders than nonathletes (Brownell, 1995). Athletes—especially those involved in sports where low body weight is considered important—are often preoccupied with body weight and shape. Athletes particularly at risk include wrestlers, distance runners, dancers, gymnasts, divers, and figure skaters. Some researchers have also theorized that the type of individual who seeks out and becomes proficient in sports because of certain personality characteristics (for example, perfectionism), may also be the type of person who is susceptible to developing eating disorders.

Athletes with eating disorders are treated in a similar manner to all individuals with eating disorders. In addition, nurses working with athletes with eating disorders must be sensitive to

- The pressure the athlete may feel to keep the disorder secret, feeling disapproval from coaches, or loss of a scholarships

- The fear the athlete has of compromised performance or participation in a sport

Nurses must work with coaches, athletic administrators, parents, and the athletes themselves to educate them on the risks of the eating disorder and the necessity of achieving nutrition goals. Nutritional rehabilitation of athletes with eating disorders may require a higher calorie intake than usual if the athlete continues to train or resumes training during treatment. Nurses must stress that athletic performance cannot be optimal if the body is not properly nourished. Athlete and therapist must view treatment of the eating disorder as first priority, and, if necessary, participation in athletics discontinued in preference to therapy.

Eating Disorders in Younger Children

Eating disorders typically begin to appear in adolescents between the ages of 14 and 16. Eating disorders in children younger than this age are less common but on the increase.

Even children as young as third or fourth grade perceive societal pressures to diet and be thin.

The term childhood eating disorders are defined as those occurring in children age 13 years and younger (Bryant-Waugh and Lask, 1995). Childhood eating disorders are clearly differenti-

ated from childhood feeding problems by the patient's preoccupation with body weight and shape and by inadequate or chaotic food intake. Anorexia nervosa in childhood is much more commonly seen than bulimia nervosa. About 25 percent of all patients with childhood eating disorders are males, compared to about 5 to 15 percent of older individuals with an eating disorder.

Because of the potential seriousness of a childhood eating disorder, treatment should be rapid and intensive. Because of the lower total body fat in children, patients with childhood onset of eating disorders are often more emaciated than adults with the disorders. Only about two-thirds of patients with such onset of eating disorders in childhood make a full recovery (Bryant-Waugh and Lask, 1995).

Nutrition therapy should allow for adequate growth. It is essential that health care providers involve the parents and family members in education and treatment. In most cases, family therapy and parental counseling are a critical element in management of childhood eating disorders.

Eating Disorders and Individuals with Diabetes

Because eating disorders affect primarily adolescents and younger adults, most individuals with both an eating disorder and diabetes have insulin-dependent, or type I diabetes. Management of an eating disorder in an individual with type I diabetes presents unique challenges for both diagnosis and management (Peveler, 1995).

Excessive dieting, bingeing, vomiting, and the misuse of laxatives and diuretics all interfere with good blood glucose control. In addition, individuals with type I diabetes have one more method of purging available to them: they can use less insulin than normal or omit their insulin dose, leading to glucose loss in the urine and rapid weight, although most of the initial weight loss is fluid.

Patients with both an eating disorder and type I

diabetes may have drastic swings in blood sugar, alternating between periods of high blood glucose levels and ketoacidosis (often severe enough to require hospitalization), and periods of low blood sugar. Traditional laboratory tests to monitor diabetes control, such as glycohemoglobin measurements, may not detect these alternating periods of high and low blood sugar. Studies also suggest that such a patient is at increased risk for developing complications of diabetes.

Fortunately, patients with type I diabetes are already more closely monitored by their family and health care providers than the general population, so eating disorders are often detected early in this population. Poor glycemic control, repeated episodes of hypoglycemia or ketoacidosis, and weight fluctuations—especially if the patient is young and a female—should clue the health provider about the possible existence of an eating disorder (Peveler, 1995).

Treatment should be closely coordinated between the eating disorder specialist and the diabetes specialist. Often the nurse can bridge the gap between the two specialists to assure continuity of care. In addition to monitoring thoughts and eating habits, health care professionals also need to monitor the patient's insulin injections and blood glucose levels. Because of the additional medical risks associated with type I diabetes, treatment that might otherwise be done on an outpatient basis may require an inpatient stay.

The next chapter reviews the role of physical activity in management of both obesity and eating disorders.

EXAM QUESTIONS

CHAPTER 11
Questions 75–81

75. A primary goal for obese individuals with type II diabetes is

    a. avoidance of dietary sugars

    b. increased dietary fiber

    c. weight loss

    d. blood sugar stabilization

76. Which of the following is considered the first line of treatment for individuals with borderline-high or high blood cholesterol levels?

    a. drug therapy

    b. diet and exercise therapy

    c. fiber therapy

    d. medical monitoring for 6 months

77. The Step-One Diet advocated by the National Cholesterol Education Program contains what percent of calories from fat?

    a. 5 percent or less

    b. 20 percent or less

    c. 25 percent or less

    d. 30 percent or less

78. According to some studies, obese children

    a. eat up to 1,000 calories more daily than nonobese children

    b. eat about 700 calories more daily than nonobese children

    c. eat about 300 calories more daily than nonobese children

    d. eat about the same number of or slightly fewer calories than nonobese children

79. About what percentage of individuals with eating disorders are male?

    a. less than 5 percent

    b. 5 to 15 percent

    c. 15 to 25 percent

    d. 25 to 35 percent

80. Which of the following groups of individuals are at greater risk of developing an eating disorder than the general population?

    a. males

    b. painters

    c. gymnasts

    d. lawyers

81. Management of an eating disorder in individuals with type I diabetes presents a unique challenge because

    a. they can omit or reduce insulin dose, leading to rapid weight loss

    b. they can vary the sugar content of their diet to obscure glycohemoglobin results

    c. they are usually younger and more resistant to treatment

    d. their parents are often overly involved and interfere with effective treatment

CHAPTER 12

INTERVENTION: PHYSICAL ACTIVITY FOR OBESITY AND EATING DISORDERS

CHAPTER OBJECTIVE

After reading this chapter, you will be able to identify the benefits of regular physical activity and to specify reasonable guidelines for exercising safely for individuals with obesity or eating disorders.

LEARNING OBJECTIVES

After studying this chapter, you will be able to

1. Identify parts of an exercise program.

2. Select appropriate type, intensity, duration, frequency, and progression of exercise for obese patients.

3. Recognize behaviors that help patients continue being physically active or exercising regularly.

4. Specify specific exercises for the severely obese person.

5. Recognize potential concerns with exercise in patients with eating disorders and identify reasonable guidelines for exercise.

INTRODUCTION

For some mildly obese individuals, physical activity may well be the only ingredient missing to achieve a healthy body weight. For example, adding a 45-minute walk three days weekly would produce a yearly weight loss of nine pounds for a person weighing 160 pounds (Walberg-Rankin, 1992). For most obese patients, however, physical activity must be combined with dietary restriction for significant weight loss (Zelasko, 1995). Combining physical activity with dietary restriction can speed up weight loss, tone muscles, and reduce risk for chronic disease.

Although regular physical activity yields many benefits, some individuals with eating disorders become overzealous with exercise and actually use it as a means of purging or to balance the perceived fattening effects of foods. This chapter will look at the benefits of exercise, discuss some specific types of exercise, and give guidelines for reasonable exercise programs for patients with obesity or eating disorders.

THE DIFFERENCE BETWEEN PHYSICAL ACTIVITY AND EXERCISE

Physical activity is any bodily movement that results in energy expenditure. Many forms of physical activity are a part of our daily routine, such as vacuuming, cleaning, gardening, lawn mowing, sweeping, shopping, painting, or walking leisurely. Exercise is a deliberate form of physical activity—a repetitive, planned activity done to improve or maintain our state of physical fitness. For many time-pressed Americans who hire for home maintenance and drive to work, however, exercise and physical activity are synonymous.

Many people believe that they must exercise vigorously and intensively to reap the benefits of exercise. Although this type of activity confers the most health benefits and provides for cardiovascular conditioning, more leisurely types of physical activity also burn calories and contribute to our overall level of physical fitness. Today experts recognize that regular moderate physical activity provides significant health benefits, even when it is done in several shorter time intervals throughout the day (Pate and colleagues, 1995).

BENEFITS OF PHYSICAL ACTIVITY

Physical activity has long been known to be beneficial for optimal health. Regular physical activity decreases death rate from all causes and from cardiovascular disease (Blair, 1995). Higher levels of leisure-time physical activity are also associated with lower rates of heart attack and better cardiorespiratory fitness (Lakka, 1994). Exercising regularly is also associated with longer life span (Lee, 1995). Physical activity has been shown to have protective effects for several chronic diseases, including high blood pressure, heart disease, type II diabetes, osteoporosis, colon cancer, and anxiety and depression (Pate, 1995).

Over the short term, physical activity maintains good muscle tone, stimulates the circulation, and aids digestion. Physical activity helps relieve stress, relaxing muscle tone and imparting a tranquilizing effect—probably partially due to the release of endorphins.

In a study of 10,269 men who graduated from Harvard College, Paffenbarger and colleagues (1993) found that moderately vigorous exercise was associated with lower overall death rates and lower death rates from coronary heart disease. In this study, beginning an exercise program reduced death risk 23 percent.

In a similar 16-year follow-up of Norwegian men, Sandvik and colleagues (1993) also found that greater levels of physical fitness are associated with lower risk of death from cardiovascular disease and death from all causes.

The first piece of good news is that people don't have to exercise at a high intensity to achieve lower levels of cardiovascular risk. In a study of 102 sedentary adult women (Duncan, 1991), women were randomly assigned to walking 4.8 kilometers daily five days at an aerobic pace, at a brisk walk, or at a leisurely stroll. Although the aerobic walking group achieved better cardiorespiratory fitness, all groups had equally favorable changes in cardiovascular risk profile. The second piece of good news is that even a midlife increase in physical activity has been shown to decrease chronic diseases and increase longevity (Paffenbarger, 1993).

Regular physical activity

- Reduces blood pressure

- Lowers levels of dangerous low-density lipoprotein (LDL) cholesterol levels

- Raises levels of protective high-density lipoprotein (HDL) cholesterol levels

- Helps stabilize blood sugar

- Burns up calories and aids in weight loss

- Relieves stress

- Tones muscles

- Helps people look and feel their best

How does physical activity help promote weight loss and weight control? When diet and exercise are combined, regular physical activity increases the rate of weight loss. Although cutting calories has the most dramatic effect of weight loss, regular physical activity can also make an important contribution.

Physical activity increases energy expenditure, so one doesn't need to cut back the number of calories so strictly, For example, if one decides to cut back 500 calories a day, or 3,500 calories a week (the amount needed to lose one pound), by adding an activity that burns 250 calories per day, one can merely cut 250 calories from the diet instead of 500. *Table 12.1* lists the approximate energy cost of many different activities. As shown in the table, the more a person weighs, the greater the energy cost of the activity.

Some individuals are afraid that physical activity will increase appetite. On the contrary, regular exercise usually decreases appetite. Dr. Jean Mayer's group (Stein, 1986) showed that food intake declines as movement is made from low- to moderate activity occupations. Physical activity also helps prevent the decline in metabolic rate that sometimes occurs with prolonged dieting.

RECOMMENDATIONS FOR LEVELS OF PHYSICAL ACTIVITY

Even when considering leisure-time physical activity, Americans rate poorly. About 27 percent of adult women in the United States and 17 percent of adult men do no type of leisure-time physical activity (Crespo, 1996). Rates of inactivity are even higher for Mexican-American men (33 percent) and women (46 percent) and black women (40 percent). Lack of time has been stated to be the main obstacle to being physically active (Pate, 1995).

The Centers for Disease Control and Prevention and the American College of Sports Medicine recently held a workshop with nationally-recognized experts to issue a public health recommendation on the types and amounts of physical activity needed for health promotion and disease prevention (Pate, 1995). Recommendations of this workshop were

> "Every U.S. adult should accumulate 30 minutes or more of moderate-intensity physical activity on most, preferably all, days of the week."

This recommendation is unique from previous recommendations in two aspects

1. It recognizes the value of less intensive forms of physical activity.

2. It acknowledges the cumulative benefits of shorter spans of physical activity over the day.

Under this new recommendation, for example, a person could walk an extra 5 minutes from a farther-away parking spot to and from work, vacuum or clean for 10 minutes after coming home from work, and go for a 10-minute bike ride with the kids after supper and still meet the goal of 30 minutes of moderate-intensity physical activity daily. For those individuals with demanding schedules, incorporating smaller amounts of physical activity throughout the day may be a more realistic approach to increasing physical activity. *Table 12.2* gives examples of intensity levels of different types of physical activities.

EXERCISING SAFELY

Most individuals can gradually incorporate more physical activity into their daily schedule. Some patients may also wish to start a regular exercise program. According to guidelines of the American College of Sports Medicine (1991), healthy men 40 years of age and younger and healthy women 50 years of age and younger do not need to consult a doctor before beginning a sensible and gradual exercise program. Older healthy individuals do not need to consult a doctor if they begin an exercise program of moderate intensity (exercise that can be comfortably continued for up to an hour at the individual's current level of fitness) and progress slowly.

TABLE 12.1 Energy Expenditure by Body Weight in Selected Physical Activities

Activity	Calories per min per lb body weight	Body weight (lb)			
		150	200	250	300
Archery	.030	4.5	6.0	7.5	9.0
Basketball	.063	9.5	12.6	15.8	18.9
Bicycling					
(5.5 mph)	.029	4.4	5.8	7.3	8.7
(9.4 mph)	.045	6.8	9.0	11.3	13.5
Canoeing (leisure)	.020	3.0	4.0	5.0	6.0
Chopping wood	.039	5.9	7.8	9.8	11.7
Cleaning house	.027	4.1	5.4	6.8	8.1
Climbing hills	.055	8.3	11.0	13.8	16.5
Cooking	.021	3.2	4.2	5.3	6.3
Dancing (slow)	.023	3.5	4.6	5.8	6.9
Dancing (fast)	.046	6.9	9.2	11.5	13.8
Digging (trenches)	.066	9.9	13.2	16.5	19.8
Field hockey	.061	9.2	12.2	15.3	18.3
Fishing	.028	4.2	5.6	7.0	8.4
Food shopping	.027	4.1	5.4	6.8	8.1
Football	.060	9.0	12.0	15.0	18.0
Golf	.039	5.9	7.8	9.8	11.7
Horse riding (trot)	.050	7.5	10.0	12.5	15.0
Ironing	.022	3.3	4.4	5.5	6.6
Lying at ease	.010	1.5	2.0	2.5	3.0
Mopping floor	.027	4.1	5.4	6.8	8.1
Mowing	.051	7.7	10.2	12.8	15.3
Painting (house)	.035	5.3	7.0	8.8	10.5
Racquetball	.096	14.4	19.2	24.0	28.8
Raking	.025	3.8	5.0	6.3	7.5
Running					
9 min/mile	.088	13.2	17.6	22.0	26.4
12 min/mile	.061	9.2	12.2	15.3	18.3
Sawing by hand	.034	5.1	6.8	8.5	10.2
Scrubbing floors	050	7.5	10.0	12.5	15.0
Sewing	.011	1.7	2.2	2.8	3.3
Sitting	.010	1.5	2.0	2.5	3.0
Skiing (downhill)	.050	7.5	10.0	12.5	15.0
Standing quietly	.012	1.8	2.4	3.0	3.6
Swimming					
Backstroke	.077	11.5	15.4	19.3	23.1
Breast stroke	.074	11.1	14.8	18.5	22.2
Crawl (fast)	.071	10.7	14.2	17.8	21.3
Crawl (slow)	.058	8.7	11.6	14.5	17.4
Table tennis	.031	4.7	6.2	7.8	9.3
Tennis	.050	7.5	10.0	12.5	15.0
Typing	.012	1.8	2.4	3.0	3.6
Volleyball	.023	3.5	4.6	5.8	6.9
Walking					
3 mph	.031	4.7	6.2	7.8	9.3
4 mph	.041	6.2	8.2	10.3	12.3
Wallpapering	.022	3.3	4.4	5.5	6.6
Weeding	.033	5.0	6.6	8.3	9.9
Window cleaning	.027	4.1	5.4	6.8	8.1

Source: Perri, M. G., Nezu, A. M., Viegener, B. J. (1992). *Improving the Long-Term Management of Obesity.* New York: John Wiley & Sons, 188–189.

TABLE 12.2 Examples of Common Physical Activities for Healthy U.S. Adults by Intensity of Effort

Light (<3.0 METs or <4 kcal•min⁻¹)	Moderate (3.0–6.0 METs or 4–7 kcal•min⁻¹)	Hard/Vigorous >6.0 METs or >7 kcal•min⁻¹
Walking slowly (strolling) (1–2 mph)	Walking, briskly (3–4 mph)	Walking, briskly uphill or with a load
Cycling, stationary (<50 W)	Cycling for pleasure or transportation (≤10 mph)	Cycling, fast or racing (>10 mph)
Swimming, slow treading	Swimming, moderate effort	Swimming, fast treading or crawl
Conditioning exercise, light stretching	Conditioning exercise, general calisthenics	Conditioning exercise, stair ergometer, ski machine
…	Racket sports, table tennis	Racket sports, singles tennis, racketball
Golf, power cart	Golf, pulling cart or carrying clubs	…
Bowling	…	…
Fishing, sitting	Fishing, standing/casting	Fishing in stream
Boating, power	Canoeing, leisurely (2.0–3.9 mph)	Canoeing, rapidly (≥4 mph)
Home care, carpet sweeping	Home care, general cleaning	Moving furniture
Mowing lawn, riding mower	Mowing lawn, power mower	Mowing lawn, hand mower
Home repair, carpentry	Home repair, painting	…

The METs (work metabolic rate/resting metabolic rate) are multiples of the resting rate of oxygen consumption during physical activity. One MET represents the approximate rate of oxygen consumption of a seated adult at rest, or about 3.5 mL•min⁻¹. The equivalent energy cost of 1 MET in kilocalories•min⁻¹ is about 1.2 for a 70-kg person, or approximately 1 kcal•kg⁻¹•hr⁻¹.

Source: Pate, R. R., Pratt, M., & Blair, S. N. (1995). Physical activity and public health: a recommendation from the Centers for Disease Control and Prevention and the American College of Sports Medicine. *Journal of the American Medical Association.* 273, 402–407.

The American College of Sports Medicine recommends that a doctor be consulted before beginning an exercise program if the patient

- Is older than 40 years for men and 50 years for women and is beginning a vigorous exercise program (a challenging regimen that tires the individual out within 20 minutes at current level of fitness)

- Has two or more risk factors for heart disease (such as high blood pressure, high blood cholesterol levels, cigarette smoking, diabetes mellitus, family history of atherosclerotic disease in parents or siblings prior to age 55)

- Has symptoms of heart disease (such as pain or pressure in the left mid-chest area, neck, shoulder, or arm during or right after exercise; shortness of breath; faintness or dizziness; palpitations, or claudication)

- Has known heart disease or other diseases that might require special attention, such as pulmonary diseases, diabetes, or bone or joint problems

While these are general guidelines, discretion should be used for each patient individually.

Patients should always be advised to start an exercise program slowly and build up gradually. Walking is a good way to start. All that is needed is a good pair of walking shoes, and patients can walk at their own pace for a comfortable distance. If pain occurs during exercise, the patient should slow down or stop. A sensible, gradual exercise program should be painless.

It's important to prepare for exercise by allowing time for stretching, a warm-up period, activity period, then a cool-down period. Stretching is important because it increases flexibility and helps prepare the body for exercise. Stretching should be done every time the patient exercises, just before warming up. Stretching should also be done after exercise to cool down. The following are some suggested stretches for various parts of the body

Neck. Stand or sit in a chair, with your arms relaxed at the sides, looking ahead. Now, slowly tilt the head to the shoulder on a slow count of 4, returning to your original position on 4 more counts. Stretch 4 times.

Sides. Stand with legs comfortably apart, toes pointing straight ahead, knees relaxed, and both arms stretched overhead. Then stretch slowly to one side on a count of 8; hold this position for a count of 10; then slowly return to the original position on a count of 8. Do this 4 times. Then stretch slowly to the other side and repeat.

Shoulders. Stand with legs comfortably apart, knees relaxed, holding a towel in your right hand. Drop the right hand over the right shoulder to the upper back. Bring the left hand under the left shoulder toward the upper back, grabbing the towel. Pull the towel slowly with the left hand. When a stretch in the shoulders is felt, hold this position for a count of 10, or about 10 seconds. Then pull the towel with the right hand, until a stretch in the shoulder is felt, Hold this position for a count of 10. Reverse the position of hands, and repeat. Do this 4 times. With practice the patient will be able to do the stretch without the towel.

Calf and Achilles tendon stretch. Stand a little more than an arm's length in front of a wall, with heels flat on the floor or ground. Place hands, at shoulder height, firmly against the wall, then slowly lean forward with legs and back straight. Try to touch shoulders and chest to the wall, turning the face to the side. When a pull in your calves is felt, hold the position for a count of 20, or about 20 seconds, keeping the heels flat on the floor. Return to the first position. Repeat this stretch 4 times.

Lower back and hamstring stretch. While seated on the floor with legs outstretched and feet together, press the backs of the legs against the floor. Slowly bend forward from the hips, keeping the back straight. Reach toward the toes and touch them if possible. Or, if the patient can't reach his feet, grasp the ankles. When the tension in the back of the legs is felt, hold the position for 10 seconds, then return to the original position. Do this stretch 4 times.

Once the patient has stretched, a warm-up period comes next. About five minutes of warming-up helps get muscles, joints, and the cardiovascular system going. For example, five minutes of easy walking helps get the body ready for further activity. A cooling-down period is important, to allow the body to return to the level it was at before exercise began. The best way to cooldown is to continue the activity at an easy pace for 5 to 10 more minutes. If walking at a brisk pace, slow down a little, swing the arms less vigorously, and take shorter steps. If swimming, slow the strokes until breathing returns to normal.

THE EXERCISE PRESCRIPTION

A discussion of physical activity can begin by having the patient estimate how much physical activity he or she currently gets. Discuss any regular exercise or activity plus day-to-day activities such as walking to work or using the stairs instead of the elevator. The health practitioner and patient can then jointly develop an exercise prescription. A trained exercise physiologist can assist in evaluating high-risk patients and developing an exercise prescription.

According to the American College of Sports Medicine (1991), an exercise prescription is a person's recommended regimen of physical activity designed to enhance fitness, promote health, and ensure safety. An exercise prescription has five main elements that must be addressed

1. Type of exercise

2. Intensity of exercise

3. Duration of exercise

4. Frequency of exercise, usually described on a weekly basis

5. Progression to more intense and longer exercise sessions

TYPE OF EXERCISE

Any regular, rhythmic exercise that works the large muscles of the body continually is good for the heart and lungs and is considered aerobic exercise. Examples of vigorous aerobic activities that definitely condition the heart and lungs if done at least 15 to 30 minutes include

- Cross-country skiing
- Ice hockey
- Jogging
- Jumping rope
- Rowing
- Running in place
- Stationary biking

Some activities that can also condition the heart and lungs if done briskly include

- Bicycling
- Basketball
- Calisthenics
- Racquetball
- Swimming
- Tennis (singles)
- Walking

Activities that can be fun, help to get you moving and use up calories but do not usually condition the heart and lungs include

- Baseball
- Bowling
- Football
- Golf
- Volleyball

Walking. Walking is enjoying a new surge of popularity largely because people of any age can walk, and it requires nothing more than a good pair of walking shoes. It uses all the major muscles of the body, can be done at varying levels, from a brisk walk to race walking, can provide just as many benefits as jogging, and produces much less strain on the knees and ankles than jogging does. Walking has also become a social event in some areas. In many larger cities, groups gather to walk through historic sections of the city or to special sites.

Nearly every program starts with a gentle pace of walking for a prescribed time or distance. For the extremely overweight person, it may be best to think in terms of blocks instead of miles. Soon it is easy to work up to a half-hour of walking, then an hour. A good measure of the speed to aim for is a walk brisk enough that the patient is breathing heavily but can still talk. Even if the patient starts out slowly, he should work up to a pace of about 4 miles per hour. Walking as little as 15 minutes a day can lead to a weight loss of up to 26 pounds a year.

Swimming. Swimming, another good exercise that can be done year-round, also helps increase the heart rate and moves all major muscles. This is often an excellent exercise for older persons because it avoids strain on the joints of the lower leg and arms. However, to be effective, swimming must be continuous and vigorous, beginning slowly at first but working up to about a half-hour. One hour of swimming will use up about 670 calories, so that every five hours of swimming equals the loss of one pound.

Cycling. Cycling is excellent for the heart, lower body muscles, and for weight loss. One can cycle nearly everywhere on the streets and side roads, or on a stationary bike in bad weather. Thirty minutes of vigorous cycling, or a speed of about 9 mph, will burn about 210 calories.

Stair-climbing. Stair-climbing is very demanding physically, and may not be good for persons who are moderately or greatly overweight. To stair-climb, a person walks up and down a flight of stairs, working up to a half hour. Climbing should be done steadily and rhythmically, resting between flights if necessary. Apparently stair-climbing uses so much energy that just climbing an extra two flights of stairs a day can lead to a weight loss of 10 to 12 pounds a year.

Stepping. This is an exercise that is well suited to persons who like to exercise in private, but it is fairly strenuous. All that is needed is a step or stool about 7 inches high. One steps up on the stool with one foot, then brings the other foot up, then steps back down with one foot, then brings the other foot down. This is a fairly strenuous exercise because stepping means lifting the total weight of the body up. It's best to start out with only four or five step-ups, then build up. Also, very heavy persons or those who are out of condition should wait until less strenuous exercises have been mastered. Working up from four or five steps to a half hour without stress is the goal.

Jogging. In many programs, jogging has been replaced with walking or alternated with walking for best results. Jogging may be too strenuous for some overweight persons; it also can lead to injuries and, of course, to dropping out of the exercise program. For others, it provides great aerobic benefits.

INTENSITY OF EXERCISE

All activity is of benefit, but to condition your heart and lungs, the activity must be brisk enough to raise heart rate and breathing somewhat. No matter what type of exercise is done, it is important to start slowly and build up gradually.

A general guideline is that the activity should make you breath a little harder, but not so hard that you couldn't talk to someone. Closer guidelines are based on heart rate. The harder the body works, the faster the heart will beat and the higher the heart rate will go. The goal is to get the heart beating in a medium zone, neither too quickly nor too slowly.

Maximum heart rate is the fastest your heart can beat. This is generally estimated by taking 220 and subtracting a person's age. The target heart rate for exercising is 60 to 75 percent of maximum heart rate *(see Table 12.3).* A beginner should aim for the lower end range of their target heart rate, while someone who has been exercising a long time should aim for the higher end of the range.

To find your pulse while exercising, place the tips of the thumb and first two fingers on either side of the throat, just below the jawbone. Here the carotid artery can be easily felt. Then, using a watch with a second hand, count the number of pulsations felt in six seconds and add a zero to that number. Another good pulse spot is the wrist. Press gently with the index and middle fingers on the thumb side of the wrist; don't use the thumb to count the pulsations because it has a pulse of its own.

DURATION OF EXERCISE

To condition the heart and lungs, the eventual goal is to have your heart beating in the target heart range for 15 to 30 continuous minutes during the active phase of exercise. For the person who isn't used to exercise, however, a few minutes in the lower end of the target heart range is a good place to start. The exercise session should always be preceded with at least a five-minute warm-up period and followed by a five-minute cool-down period

Exercise Session

Warm-up	5 minutes
Exercise	15 to 30 minutes
Cool down	5 minutes
TOTAL TIME	25 to 40 minutes

TABLE 12.3 Target Heart Rates

Age in years	Target Zone (beats per minute) (60–75% of maximum)	Average Maximum Heart Rate 100% (beats per minute)
20	120–150	200
25	117–146	195
30	114–142	190
35	111–138	185
40	108–135	180
45	105–131	175
50	102–127	170
55	99–123	165
60	96–120	160
65	93–116	155
70	90–113	150

Source: National Institutes Fact Sheet on Exercise.

FREQUENCY OF EXERCISE

You don't have to exercise every day to reap the benefits of exercise. Exercise physiologists now advise that you exercise three to five times weekly. Even people who exercise only three times weekly will be amazed at how much better they will feel. Regular exercise three to five times weekly will firm up muscles, increase energy level, burn off extra calories, and reduce stress and tension.

PROGRESSION

With any new exercise routine, a person should start slowly and build up gradually. As a person continues to exercise, the exercise becomes easier and intensity and duration of the exercise session can be gradually increased.

How fast to progress with more vigorous and longer exercise sessions depends on many factors, such as a person's age, health status, preferences and goals. Most people can gradually progress to a regular exercise routine of appropriate duration and intensity over six to eight weeks. Very overweight individuals and individuals who have not exercised in a long time may progress slower. Individuals who are in better physical condition to start with may progress faster. If the patient experiences stiffness or soreness after exercise, he or she is progressing too fast.

STICKING WITH IT

Getting established in an exercise routine isn't always easy. However, there are some ways the nurse can help the patient stick with it and eventually lead a more active life. The trick is to make activity a regular part of life, not merely a short-term effort.

Encourage them to try to think of ways to be more active at work, at home, and in other settings. Some examples include parking farther away from a store so that one will have to walk a longer distance. Other measures, like reducing television time and substituting other activities, may help get some "couch potatoes" up and out of the deadly easy chair in front of the TV.

Another good idea is to search out local swimming pools and gymnasiums and the local YMCA and YWCA. Use facilities that are conveniently located near home or work.

Having good companionship during exercise can also be a great help, and in fact may be the key to keeping a patient active. For some persons, participating in a group activity, such as aerobics class, is the strongest factor that compels them to keep exercising. Finding a good walking companion or a group can help turn an ordinary brisk walk into an adventure. Social support is extremely important.

Finally, the activity has to be enjoyable or it stands a good chance of being dropped. Once a person becomes proficient in an activity and finds that he enjoys it, for companionship or better health, it is likely that it will become a permanent addition to a healthier life.

EXERCISES FOR SEVERELY OBESE PERSONS

For the person who is extremely overweight, it may be nearly impossible to jump right into a typical exercise program (Foss, 1984). A more cautious approach, starting with a thorough checkup, is best. At Johns Hopkins Hospital, obese patients start with a sitting exercise program in which patients do exercises in a chair with no arms, then add a 5-minute walk every day. These patients are warned against participating in exercises such as jogging, rope jumping, weight-lifting, climbing stairs, one-legged exercises, or competitive sports, all of which can be dangerous to their health. Patients begin with three months or more of sitting exercises and walking, then advance to swimming, walking, or exercises on a stationary bicycle.

Some examples of beginning sitting exercises might include the following

Seated jumping jacks. Swing arms overhead, touching the backs of the hands to each other, simultaneously moving the feet as far apart as possible. Return to starting position. Start with three repetitions, and work up to 10.

Side-stretchers. Raise left hand overhead with palm toward the ceiling. Place right hand on the hip or the arm of the chair, and lean to the

right as far as possible. Stretch out four times. Now reverse the procedure, raising the right hand and placing the left hand on the hip, leaning to the left and stretching.

This gentle and gradual approach to exercise helps very overweight persons stick with it. As they cut down on their calories, good results are seen.

EXERCISE AND PATIENTS WITH EATING DISORDERS

While regular physical activity yields many benefits, some individuals with eating disorders overexercise because of a perceived disturbance in body image, to balance the perceived fattening effects of certain foods, or to help burn calories consumed in binge episodes. Nutritional therapy for patients with eating disorders includes adjusting net calorie balance for weight gain. Because of the positive health benefits or exercise, however, exercise should not be entirely forbidden but rather kept to reasonable limits.

For most individuals, 20 to 30 minutes of regular aerobic exercise three to five times weekly is reasonable (Reichert, 1993). Exercise beyond this level should be questioned.

As discussed in chapter eleven, athletes, especially female athletes, are at increased risk for developing eating disorders. If the individual is exercising intensively to remain or regain competitiveness, calories expended in physical activity can be estimated and balanced with equivalent increases in dietary intake. If the individual is unable or unwilling to make the necessary dietary adjustments to accommodate increased exercise, the individual may need to discontinue the sport or activity in favor of treatment.

The final chapter of this book describes techniques for long-term weight maintenance, recovery, and prevention of obesity and eating disorders.

EXAM QUESTIONS

CHAPTER 12
Questions 82–91

82. For a person weighing 160 pounds, adding a 45-minute walk three days weekly would produce a yearly weight loss of about how many pounds?

    a. 5

    b. 9

    c. 15

    d. 20

83. Physical activity has been shown to help prevent or treat which of the following chronic diseases?

    a. high blood pressure

    b. osteoporosis

    c. heart disease

    d. all of the above

84. Which of the following is often true regarding physical activity and appetite?

    a. Physical activity reduces appetite.

    b. Physical activity increases appetite.

    c. Physical activity has no effect on appetite.

    d. Greater appetite reduces physical activity levels.

85. Which of the following reflects new recommendations regarding levels of physical activity?

    a. Adults should accumulate 30 minutes or more of moderate-intensity physical activity on most or all days of the week.

    b. Adults should accumulate 60 minutes or more of moderate-intensity physical activity on most or all days of the week.

    c. Adults should exercise intensively about 30 minutes three or four days weekly.

    d. Adults should exercise intensively 60 minutes or more three or four days weekly.

86. How often should stretching be done in an exercise prescription?

    a. before every exercise session

    b. before every other exercise session

    c. before and after every exercise session

    d. after every exercise session

87. Which of the following is not an element of the exercise prescription?

    a. type of exercise

    b. cycle of exercise

    c. intensity of exercise

    d. duration of exercise

88. Which of the following activities best conditions the heart and lungs

    a. baseball

    b. golf

    c. cross-country skiing

    d. bowling

89. To have the greatest chance of continuing to exercise regularly, individuals should choose an activity that is

    a. vigorous

    b. enjoyable

    c. inexpensive

    d. solitary and can be done alone

90. Severely obese individuals might begin an exercise program with which type of exercises?

    a. sitting exercises

    b. standing exercises

    c. jogging

    d. swimming

91. Reasonable guidelines for exercise in most patients with eating disorders would be

    a. 10 minutes of vigorous activity five days weekly

    b. 20 to 30 minutes of regular aerobic exercise three to five times weekly

    c. 50 to 60 minutes of regular aerobic exercise four to five times weekly

    d. discontinue exercise until the eating disorder is resolved

CHAPTER 13

EVALUATION: WEIGHT MAINTENANCE, RECOVERY AND PREVENTION

CHAPTER OBJECTIVE

After reading this chapter, you will be able to identify factors that help patients achieve life-long changes for weight maintenance.

LEARNING OBJECTIVES

After studying this chapter, you will be able to

1. Specify components of a comprehensive program that increase the likelihood of maintaining a stable body weight loss long-term.

2. Recognize strategies in preventing relapse after weight loss.

3. Identify strategies for long-term recovery from an eating disorder.

4. Indicate ways to promote primary prevention of obesity and eating disorders in the general population.

INTRODUCTION

For an obese patient, losing weight takes great effort and vigilance. For a person with an eating disorder, gaining weight or stabilizing weight and eating behavior takes equally as much effort and vigilance. For those who reach this stage, however, the battle is not over. The second, and perhaps more difficult, step is maintenance of

weight and preventing relapse. This chapter will review components of care that promote long-term recovery, weight maintenance, and relapse prevention for persons with obesity or an eating disorder. Finally, the chapter will review prevention strategies for obesity and eating disorders in the general population.

SUCCESSFUL WEIGHT MAINTENANCE AFTER WEIGHT LOSS

A Continuous Care Model

Few studies evaluate maintenance of weight loss over the long term. Of the few that do, results show that most individuals regain most of the weight lost (Perri, 1992). Physiological processes such as lowered metabolic weight and altered body chemistry can work against efforts to maintain weight loss. Feeling continually restricted and following a rigid diet over the long term can also increase the likelihood of relapse.

Almost all patients who have lost weight relapse from strict adherence to their diet and exercise routine at some point. Because of this strong possibility of relapse after weight loss, Dr. Michael Perri, a psychologist at the University of Florida in Gainesville, proposes a continuous care model for obesity management. The model asserts that obesity is a chronic condition that requires long-term care. After initial treatment for obesity, Perri (1993) advocates comprehensive programs that combine continued professional contact, skills training in relapse prevention, social support, and exercise to enhance long-term weight maintenance.

Elements of a Successful Weight Maintenance Program

Realistic Goals The first step of setting realistic weight maintenance goals is to set realistic weight loss goals. If the nurse has helped the patient set realistic goals for weight loss, then maintaining those goals over the long-term will be easier. If a woman who is 5'4" tall and weighed 200 pounds at the beginning of treatment set a goal weight of 120 pounds, maintenance of that weight would be extremely difficult physiologically and psychologically. If her initial goal weight was to lose 20 pounds, or 10 percent of body weight, maintenance of those 20 pounds over the long-term would be easier, though still an accomplishment.

Patients should not expect perfection in weight maintenance or complete adherence to a dietary or exercise program. Everyone's weight fluctuates, and everyone occasionally indulges in high-calorie foods or gets off their exercise routine at some point. Individuals who have lost weight should expect that these things will happen and plan in advance how to handle them. The important thing is not to let such events derail the entire weight maintenance effort, but to get right back on track again. Grilo and Brownell (1993) state that successful goals for weight maintenance are

1. Specific (i.e., begin a walking program on Tuesday morning before work, rather than begin a walking program sometime next week).

2. Broken down into short- and long-term goals (such as walking 5 minutes longer each day toward an eventual goal of walking 45 minutes four times weekly).

3. Require constant evaluation, looking at progress and problems.

Grilo and Brownell also state that a person trying to maintain weight loss should try to keep sight of the many benefits, such as improved health, a higher level of fitness, more confidence, greater well-being, and feeling and looking better.

A Life-Long Eating Plan

Adhering to a very restricted and rigid diet over the longterm is difficult at a minimum and almost impossible for some people. Following a balanced diet that is low in fats and high in carbohydrates during the weight-loss phase teaches diet principles that promote long-term weight maintenance.

Diets that are low in fats and high in complex carbohydrates and fiber offer a greater volume of food at a lower calorie level, providing a greater degree of satiety and feeling of fullness and helping to prevent overeating (Anderson, 1987). When an individual usually follows such a diet, an occasional fat- and calorie-laden food will not have much impact on weight.

Continued Professional Contact

Some professionals have tried providing "booster" sessions after weight loss to review and reinforce diet and exercise concepts learned during the weight-loss phase. There are often three to six such sessions held one to three months apart. After reviewing the literature, Perri (1992) concluded that such sessions are not as effective as they could be. Sessions may have been too far apart, with too little professional contact.

To be most effective, Perri states that professional contact must be frequent and geared specifically toward weight maintenance. Maintaining weight loss brings a whole new set of challenges compared to weight loss. Therefore, therapist contact should focus on helping the patient anticipate high-risk situations, solve problems, and develop coping skills to prevent relapse. As an alternative to conventional appointments, Perri suggests having the patient telephone the therapist and mail in written activity and eating records.

Perri compared weight maintenance of six groups of subjects to determine the impact of intensive and continued professional contact. The first three groups had no continued professional contact and received (1) only diet instruction; (2) diet instruction plus behavior modification instruction, and (3) diet and behavior modification instruction plus training in relapse prevention. The next three groups had the same initial treatment as the above three groups but also had continued professional contact for six months after weight loss.

The groups that had training in all three areas—diet, behavior modification, and relapse prevention—plus continued professional contact had the best weight maintenance of all groups and maintained most of their initial weight loss at both the six-month and 12-month follow-up.

Social Support

Perri (1992) also compared the effects of long-term contact with a therapist or a peer support group on weight maintenance. Subjects in the peer support groups met bi-weekly. Other subjects had contact with their therapist on a bi-weekly basis. At 18 months after weight loss, both methods improved maintenance of weight loss compared to conventional behavior therapy with no continued peer or professional contact.

Close family and friends of the patient can also help, or hinder, the patient's weight-maintenance efforts. From the beginning, it's important for the patient to have the support of those around him or her. Without the support of family members or significant others, eating can be easily sabotaged. Here are some ways to enlist cooperation

- Invite the patient's spouse to a counseling session, especially if he or she does most of the shopping for and preparation of foods.

- Ask for the family member's support, explain

the gradual but lasting changes that can be made in the patient's diet, and keep them informed of the patient's progress.

- Ask family to help the patient cut down his or her exposure to the problem foods, for example, by not keeping these foods around or keeping them out of sight.

- Work with a family member if he or she has similar family needs.

- If there are children at home, ask them to help with selection and preparation of foods.

- For anyone who lives alone, particularly older persons, have them ask friends for encouragement and support.

Help patients prepare for possible problems with the people they live with and remind them to ask, not demand, their help.

Regular Physical Activity

Just as physical activity may well be the only ingredients missing from a weight-loss program, it may also be the missing ingredient for successful weight maintenance. In fact, continuing exercise is one of the best predictors of successful weight maintenance.

In one study, only those subjects who continued exercising regularly maintained most of their weight loss after two years (Van Dale, 1990). In Perri's studies (1992), subjects in a weight-maintenance program who had continued therapist contact, behavioral training, social support, and 180 minutes of aerobic exercise weekly maintained 99 percent of their initial weight loss at the 18-month follow-up.

While following a rigid diet day after day requires constant vigilance, walking 30 minutes three to four times weekly is a much easier and more controllable activity for most people. Without making any conscientious changes in diet, walking one mile every day would help most individuals lose about 14 pounds a year.

Skills For Preventing Relapse

In the weight maintenance phase, the therapist must help the patient identify and cope with barriers to weight maintenance. The problems the patient encounters in the weight-maintenance phase are different from those in the weight-loss phase. The therapist and the patient must problem-solve together, and prevent minor slips from becoming major relapses.

In the relapse cycle, an individual confronts some type of high-risk situation that challenges eating control. The situation could be a social event, an argument with a spouse, a stressful day, or any of a number of situations that trigger overeating. With no coping skills, the individual can lose control over his or her eating. This loss of control undermines the individual's confidence and self-esteem. Thoughts like "I really blew it this time, so I might as well wait until next week to get back on track" or "I'll never be able to keep my weight off" become self-fulfilling. One lapse leads to another, and pretty soon the patient abandons all control, falls into total relapse, and regains of much of the initial weight loss.

Perri (1992) and Brownell (1992) both outline several strategies to help prevent relapse. First, the therapist should help the patient identify high-risk situations that could lead to loss of control over eating. The therapist might ask the patient to keep a record of high-risk situations over a few week's time, to list situations that have triggered loss of control in the past, or to imagine a likely high-risk situation.

Next, the therapist must help the patient develop skills for coping with his or her high-risk situations. This might mean bringing a lower-calorie dish to a social gathering, planning ahead what to order at a restaurant, being assertive with friends or family, keeping certain foods out of the house, making a list of alternative activities when the urge to splurge strikes, or even preplanning a splurge. Patients may also want to have a plan of action in place if a certain amount of weight is regained— say three to five pounds.

The therapist should encourage the patient to practice and evaluate coping strategies. Often times maintenance groups go out to a restaurant together or schedule a potluck meal to review coping strategies. Practicing these strategies builds self-confidence and gives the individual a feeling of control.

Finally, the therapist must help the patient counter negative thoughts when he or she loses control.

RECOVERY FROM AN EATING DISORDER

Although the nutritional inadequacies and weight deficits associated with eating disorders can be restored in fairly short time periods with vigilance and cooperation of the patient, it takes much longer to change underlying thoughts and feelings about body image, dieting, and food. With regular therapy, some patients with eating disorders can make a full recovery in one to two years. For others, eight to ten years of therapy are needed, with the average time period being about five years.

Therapy is most effective when there is continuity of care, with the same therapist working with the patient over the short and long term, and when family members or significant others are involved, if needed (Fichter, 1995). During periods of crisis or relapse, therapy sessions may need to be more often. If an impasse occurs, consultation with a second therapist may be necessary.

Ongoing therapy to help treat eating disorders and prevent relapse involves guided exposure to risky situations while the patient practices coping or response strategies (Tuschen and Bents, 1995). During long-term therapy, cues in the patient's usual environment that might provoke relapse are anticipated and simulated. Dysfunctional thoughts and feelings are anticipated ahead of time and alternative thoughts and reactions are substituted, providing the patient an opportunity to practice new skills. As therapy continues, any problem situation is viewed as an opportunity to practice new coping skills.

Exposure to "Forbidden" Foods

Patients are gradually confronted with foods they considered to be forbidden or fattening in a controlled setting that becomes gradually more varied. Patients should taste the food and verbalize its smell, taste, consistency, and appearance to desensitize themselves to the food.

Exposure to Binge Food Triggers of Binge Eating

Certain foods or negative thoughts or feelings that trigger episodes of binge-eating are also confronted. Over time, prolonged exposure to a variety of binge foods takes place, desensitizing the patient to their effects. The therapist can help the patient problem-solve to devise strategies to counter negative thoughts and feelings that trigger binges. This might include assertiveness training or working on interpersonal relationships.

Exposure to Body Shape

Patients with eating disorders usually do not like to look at themselves. Exposure therapy to body shape involves the patient viewing himself or herself in a full-length mirror. This can be done at home or during therapy in a variety of clothing styles.

These sessions are designed to help patients recognize and accept the attractive and less attractive parts of their bodies the way they are.

Exposure to Body Weight

Exposure to body weight is similar to exposure to body shape. Patients can weigh themselves under varying conditions to desensitize themselves to negative thoughts and feelings and decrease their anxieties surrounding body weight. Patients also learn that weight fluctuations throughout the day are normal.

Addressing Body Image Disturbances

Correcting underlying disturbances in body image should be a primary goal of long-term therapy for eating disorders. Unless the nurse and other health professionals address disturbances in body image during therapy, the patient with eating disorders is likely to have reoccurring symptoms and relapse (Rosen, 1995). Other psychological variables such as psychopathy, stress, and family dysfunction are also associated with recurrent eating disorder symptoms but not nearly to the extent predicted by body image disturbance.

PREVENTION OF OBESITY AND EATING DISORDERS

Unfortunately, prevention of obesity and eating disorders is not nearly as simple as prevention of small pox or polio, where a single causative agent is responsible and where one preventative measure works almost universally. Obesity and eating disorders are complex conditions that resist treatment, let alone prevention.

Experts define prevention efforts on three levels (Fairburn, 1995; Stunkard, 1995). Primary prevention aims at preventing (or delaying) the onset of new cases of the disease. Primary prevention for obesity or eating disorders means preventing people from becoming obese or developing an eating disorder. Primary prevention efforts are geared to the general public.

Secondary prevention aims to decrease the rate of established cases of the disease. For obesity and eating disorders, secondary prevention efforts would be geared to getting the obese person or the persons with an eating disorder in to seek help.

Secondary prevention also aims to prevent a further worsening of the condition. For obese individuals, this means preventing further weight gain. Secondary prevention efforts increase awareness and are geared to individuals with or at risk for the disease.

Tertiary prevention aims at limiting disability or impairments associated with a disease and is really a part of treatment. For obese patients, tertiary prevention means decreasing the progression to more severe levels of obesity or decreasing the risk of obesity-related problems such as high blood pressure, type II diabetes, or cardiovascular disease. More patients recover fully from eating disorders than from obesity, so tertiary prevention is not always necessary. However, in the smaller proportion of patients for which an eating disorder becomes a lifelong battle, tertiary prevention aims at reducing the mortality and morbidity associated with the disorder. Tertiary prevention efforts are geared to individuals with the disease.

Primary prevention for eating disorders should be geared to school-aged children, adolescents, and college-age students, since eating disorders usually first appear in these age ranges. Primary prevention programs should target reduction in the behaviors that can trigger eating disorders: dieting and diet-related behaviors such as bingeing, vomiting, and misuse of laxatives. Primary prevention programs for eating disorders should also teach individuals to resist the pressures from the media to be overly thin and to resist peerpressure to diet or engage in harmful diet-related behaviors.

Secondary prevention for eating disorders involves educating the public about general features and nature of eating disorders so that they can be recognized and treated early. Many times individuals wait to seek help for eating disorders. Obstacles to seeking help include (Fairburn, 1995)

- The disorder is not viewed as a problem. This is especially true for those with anorexia ner-

vosa; thus a concerned significant other is often the one persuading the individual with the disorder to seek help.

- The individual hopes the disorder will go away on its own.

- The individual believes the eating disorder is not severe enough to merit professional help, or that they do not deserve professional help.

- The individual does not want others to know they have a problem, since feelings of shame, guilt, and secrecy are common, especially among those with bulimia nervosa.

- Individuals have difficulty telling their doctor about their problem. Often the patient will present with a related problem instead, such as menstrual irregularity, gastrointestinal problems, or depression.

- Individuals fear treatment and weight gain.

- Individuals do not have the financial resources to pay for treatment.

Because of the high rate of obesity among the U.S. population, education programs aimed at obesity prevention will probably be working at all three levels of prevention simultaneously. Six outcome measures have been identified for population-based approaches to preventing obesity (Food and Nutrition Board, 1995)

1. Reduce the prevalence of obesity in the general population.

2. Reduce average body weight in the U.S. population.

3. Improve nutritional intake, eating habits, exercise, and health-related activities.

4. Improve knowledge, attitudes, and norms regarding nutrition, weight, eating habits, and exercise habits.

5. Decrease rates of co-existing problems, such as hypertension and diabetes.

6. Make public policy and environmental changes

to promote weight reduction.

Examples of population-based obesity prevention programs include

Family-based programs involve educating the family on food purchasing, food presentation, and modeling to influence eating behavior of the entire family and prevent obesity in children in the family.

School-based programs emphasize education about nutrition and exercise for health promotion. The school environment is also included in school-base programs, since children eat one to two meals daily in schools.

Work-site-based programs are health promotion programs that can reach a large number of people at a low cost. Work-site programs include education on nutrition, exercise, weight control. The work-place cafeteria may participate and change foods selection. Weigh-in contests between groups of employees or departments can also be used.

Communitywide programs target the entire population within a specific community. Communitywide weight-control programs

have usually been part of a larger program aimed at a related disorder, for example, cardiovascular disease prevention programs.

Although all these types of prevention approaches have admirable goals, research evaluating the effects of such programs yield disappointing results (Fairburn, 1995; Stunkard, 1995; and Food and Nutrition Board, 1995). Education and knowledge may be necessary for change, but it seems that they are not the only elements needed.

If complex and powerful sociocultural factors have contributed to the rising incidence of obesity and eating disorders in the past few decades, then it may be these same factors that we need to modify to help prevent obesity and eating disorders.

In the past few decades Americans have become more sedentary, have a greater variety of high-calorie foods available, and place increasing emphasis and value on thinness.

If obesity and eating disorders are to be truly prevented, the media, the fashion industry, the food industry, the medical industry, government policy, society, and ultimately, we ourselves, must change to adopt healthier lifestyles, values, and choices.

EXAM QUESTIONS

CHAPTER 13
Questions 92–100

92. A model that asserts that obesity is a chronic condition that requires long-term care is called

    a. the chronic condition model of obesity follow-up

    b. the intensive care model of obesity treatment

    c. the continuous care model for obesity management

    d. the monitoring model for obesity management

93. What percentage of patients who have lost weight relapse from strict adherence to their diet and exercise routine at some point during maintenance?

    a. 35 percent

    b. 50 percent

    c. 75 percent

    d. almost 100 percent

94. One element of a successful weight-maintenance program is

    a. reading of diet-related books

    b. regular review of weight-loss strategies

    c. continued professional contact

    d. daily weight charting

95. The support of close family and friends should be enlisted in the patient's weight maintenance efforts because

    a. they may also be overweight and may need diet guidance

    b. a diet can be easily sabotaged by family and friends

    c. family and friends can provide valuable insight into the patient's diet adherence

    d. the patient may be more open to diet suggestions from family and friends

96. Which takes longer to change in the patient with an eating disorder?

    a. nutritional status

    b. weight deficit

    c. food-related behavior

    d. thoughts and feelings about body image and food

97. Ongoing therapy to help treat patients with eating disorders involves

    a. maintaining a strict diet plan

    b. guided exposure to risky eating situations

    c. gradual attainment of ideal body weight

    d. guided reestablishment of all significant relationships

98. Secondary prevention of obesity and eating disorders aims to

    a. prevent the onset of new cases of obesity or eating disorders

    b. decrease the rate of established cases of obesity or eating disorders

    c. limit disability or impairments associated with obesity or eating disorders

    d. secondary prevention of obesity and eating disorders is not possible

99. Primary prevention programs for eating disorders should be geared toward which of the following populations?

    a. elderly individuals

    b. obese individuals

    c. adolescents

    d. middle-aged individuals

100. Population-based obesity prevention programs include which of the following?

    a. family-based programs

    b. school-based programs

    c. communitywide programs

    d. all of the above

BIBLIOGRAPHY

Abraham, S., Collins, G., and Nordsieck, L. (1971). Relationship of childhood weight status to morbidity in adults. *HSMHA Health Reports,* 86, 273–384.

Albright, A. L., & Stern, J. S. (1995). Energy intake and body weight. In K. D. Brownell, & C. G. Fairburn, (Eds.). *Eating disorders and obesity,* (pp. 27–31). New York: The Guilford Press.

American College of Sports Medicine. (1991). *Guidelines for exercise testing and prescription* (4th ed.). Philadelphia: Lea and Febiger.

American Diabetes Association, position statement. (1996). Nutrition recommendations and principles for people with diabetes mellitus. *Diabetes Care.* 19 (Suppl 1), S16–19.

American Diabetes & Dietetic Associations. (1988). *Eating Healthy Foods.* Alexandria, VA: The American Diabetes Association, Chicago, IL: The American Dietetic Association.

American Diabetes & Dietetic Associations. (1996). *Exchange Lists for Weight Management.* Alexandria, VA: The American Diabetes Association, Chicago, IL: The American Dietetic Association.

American Dietetic Association. (1994). Position of The American Dietetic Association: Nutrition intervention in the treatment of anorexia nervosa, bulimia nervosa, and binge eating. *Journal of the American Dietetic Association.* 94, 902–907.

American Dietetic Association. (1989). Position of the American Dietetic Association: Optimal weight as a health promotion strategy. Journal of the *American Dietetic Association* 89, 1814–17.

American Heart Association (1997, October 10). *Fenfluramine/phentermine media advisory.* Dallas: Author.

American Psychiatric Association. (1994). *Diagnostic and statistical manual of mental disorders, 4th edition.* Washington, D.C.: American Psychiatric Association.

Andersen, A. E. (1995). Eating disorders in males. In K. D. Brownell, & C. G. Fairburn, (Eds.). *Eating disorders and obesity,* (pp. 177–182). New York: The Guilford Press.

Anderson, H. G. (1994). Regulation of food intake. In M. E. Shils, J. A. Olson, & M. Shike. *Modern nutrition in health and disease,* (8th edition), (pp. 524–536). Philadelphia: Lea & Febiger.

Anderson, J. W. & Gustafson, N. J. (1987). Dietary fiber in disease prevention and treatment. *Comprehensive Therapy* 13, 43–53.

Anderson, J. W. & Gustafson, N. J. (1988). Hypocholesterolemic effects of oat and bean products. *American Journal of Clinical Nutrition* 48 (suppl), 749S–753S.

Ashley, F. & Kannel, W. (1974). Relation of weight change to changes in atherogenic traits: The Framingham Study. *Journal of Chronic Diseases* 27, 103–114.

Astrup, A., Buemann, B., Toubro, S., Ranneries, C., & Raben, A. (1996). Low resting metabolic rate in subjects predisposed to obesity: a role for thyroid status. *American Journal of Clinical Nutrition* 63, 879–883.

Atkinson, R. L. (1989). Low and very low calorie diets. *Medical Clinics of North America* 73, 203–215.

Atkinson, R. L., & Hubbard, V. S. (1994). Report on the NIH Workshop on Pharmacologic Treatment of Obesity. *American Journal of Clinical Nutrition* 60, 153–156.

Ballor, D. L., McCarthy, J. P., & Wilterdink, E. J. (1990). Exercise intensity does not affect composition of diet- and exercise-induced body mass loss. *American Journal of Clinical Nutrition* 51, 142–6.

Beaumont, P. J. V., & Touyz, S. W. (1995). The nutritional management of anorexia and bulimia nervosa. In K. D. Brownell, & C. G. Fairburn, (Eds.). *Eating disorders and obesity,* (pp. 306–312). New York: The Guilford Press.

Bierman, E. & Brunzell, J. D. (1992). Obesity and atherosclerosis. In P. Bjorntorp & B. N. Brodoff (Eds.), *Obesity* (pp. 512–516). Philadelphia: J. B. Lippincott Co.

Bjorntorp, P. (1991). Metabolic implications of body fat distribution. *Diabetes Care* 14, 1132–43.

Bjorvell, H. & Rossner, S. (1992). A ten year follow-up of weight change in severely obese subjects treated in a behavioral modification program. *International Journal of Obesity* 16, 623–625.

Blackburn, G. L., & Kanders, B. S. (1987). Medical evaluation and treatment of the obese patient with cardiovascular disease. *American Journal of Cardiology* 60, 55G–58G.

Blair, S. N., Kohl, H. W. III, Barlow, C. E., Paffenbarger, R. S. Jr., Gibbons, L. W., & Macera C. A. (1995). Changes in physical fitness and all-cause mortality. *Journal of the American Medical Association.* 273, 1093–1098.

Blundell, J. E. (1990). Appetite disturbance and the problems of overweight. *Drugs* 39 (Suppl 3), 1–19.

Bowen, D. J., Tomoyasu, N. & Cauce, A. M. (1991). The triple threat: a discussion of gender, class, and race difference in weight. *Women's Health* 17, 123–43.

Bray, G. A. (1979). Obesity in America: An overview of the Second Fogarty International Center Conference on Obesity. *International Journal of Obesity* 3, 363–375.

Bray, G. A. (1985). Complications of obesity. *Annals of Internal Medicine* 103, 1052–62.

Bray, G. A. (1985). Obesity: Definition, diagnosis, and disadvantages. *Australian Journal of Medicine,* 142 (Suppl 7), S2–S8.

Bray, G. A. (1990). Exercise and obesity. In C. Bouchard, R. J. Shepard, T. Stephans, et al. (Eds.), *Exercise, fitness, and health,* (pp. 497–510). Champaign, IL: Human Kinetics.

Brown, P. J., & Konner, M. (1987). An anthropological perspective on obesity. *Annals of the New York Academy of Science,* 499, 29–46.

Brownell, K. D. (1995). Eating disorders in athletes. In K. D. Brownell, & C. G. Fairburn, (Eds.). *Eating disorders and obesity,* (pp. 191–198). New York: The Guilford Press.

Brownell, K. D. (1992). Relapses and the treatment of obesity. In T. A. Wadden & Van Itallie, T. B. (Eds.), *Treatment of the Seriously Obese Patient.,* (pp. 437–55). New York: The Guildford Press.

Brownell, K. D., & Fairburn, C. G., (Eds.) (1995). *Eating disorders and obesity.* New York: The Guilford Press.

Brownell, K. D. & Stunkard, A. J. (1980). Physical activity in the development and control of obesity. In. A. L. Stunkard (Ed.), *Obesity,* (pp. 300–324). Philadelphia: Saunders.

Bruch, H. (1978). *The golden cage: The enigma of anorexia nervosa.* New York: Random House.

Bryant-Waugh, R., & Lask, B. (1995). Childhood-onset eating disorders. In K. D. Brownell, & C. G. Fairburn, (Eds.). *Eating disorders and obesity,* (pp. 183–187).

Butrum, R. R., Clifford, C. K. & Lanza E. (1988). NCI dietary guidelines: Rationale. *American Journal of Clinical Nutrition* 48, 888–891.

Callaway, C. W., & Pemberton, C. (1985). Relationship of basal metabolic rates to meal-eating patterns. In: J. Hirsch & T. B. Van Itallie, (Eds.), *Recent advances in obesity research. Proceedings of the 4th International Congress on Obesity,* (pp. 50A). London: Libbey.

Cannistra, L.B., Davis, S.M., & Bauman, A.G. (1997). Valvular heart disease associated with dexfenfluramine [Letter to the editor]. *New England Journal of Medicine, 337,* 636.

Case, R. B., Heller, S. S., Case, N. B., et. al. (1985). Multicenter Post-Infraction Research Group: Type A behavior and survival after acute myocardial infarction. *New England Journal of Medicine* 312, 737–741.

Connolly, H.M., Crary, J.L., McGoon, M.D., Hensrud, D.D., Edwards, B.S., Edwards, W.D., & Schaff, H.V. (1997). Valvular heart disease associated with fenfluramine-phentermine. *New England Journal of Medicine, 337,* 581–588.

Cooper, Z. (1995). The development and maintenance of eating disorders. In K. D. Brownell, & C. G. Fairburn, (Eds.). *Eating disorders and obesity,* (pp. 199–206). New York: The Guilford Press.

Crespo, C. J., Keteyian, S. J., Heath, G. W., & Sempos, C. T. (1996). Leisure-time physical activity among US adults: results from the Third National Health and Nutrition Examination Survey. *Archives of Internal Medicine.* 156, 93–99.

Curfman, G.D. (1997). Diet pills redux [Editorial]. *New England Journal of Medicine, 337,* 629–630.

DeFronzo, R. A. & Ferrannini, E. (1991). Insulin resistance: A multifaceted syndrome responsible for NIDDM, obesity, hypertension, dyslipidemia, and atherosclerotic cardiovascular disease. *Diabetes Care* 14, 173–94.

de Gennes, C. (1993). Osteoarticular pathology and massive obesity. *Reviews of Practice* 43, 1924–1929.

Despres, J. P., Moorjani, S., & Lupien, P. J. (1990). Regional distribution of body fat, plasma, lipoproteins, and cardiovascular disease. *Arteriosclerosis* 10, 497–511.

de Zwaan, M., Nutzinger, D. O. & Schoenbeck, G. (1992). Binge eating in overweight women. *Comprehensive Psychiatry* 33, 256–61.

de Zwaan, M., & Mitchell, J. E. (1993). Medical complications of anorexia nervosa and bulimia nervosa. In A. S. Kaplan & P. E. Garfinkel, (Eds.). *Medical issues and the eating disorders: the interface.* (pp.1–16). New York: Brunner/Mazel Publishers.

Dietz, W. (1992). Childhood obesity. In P. Bjorntorp & B. N. Brodoff (Eds.). *Obesity,* (pp. 606–609). Philadelphia: J. B. Lippincott Co.

Duncan, J. J., Gordon, N. F. & Scott, C. B. (1991). Women walking for health and fitness: How much is enough? *Journal of the American Medical Association* 266, 3295–3299.

Dwyer, J. T. (1992). Treatment of obesity: Conventional programs and fad diets. In P. Bjorntorp & B. N. Brodoff, (Eds.). *Obesity,* (pp. 662–667). Philadelphia: J. B. Lippincott Co.

Eckel, R. H. (1992). Insulin resistance: and adaptation for weight maintenance. *Lancet.* 340, 1452–1453.

Eliahou, H. E., Shechter, P., & Blare, A. (1992). Hypertension in obesity. In P. Bjorntorp & B. N. Brodoff, (Eds). *Obesity* (pp. 532–39). Philadelphia: J. B. Lippincott Co.

Everhart, J. E., Pettitt, D. J., & Bennett, P. H. (1992). Duration of obesity increases the incidence of NIDDM. *Diabetes* 41, 235–40.

Fairburn, C. G. (1995). The prevention of eating disorders. In K. D. Brownell, & C. G. Fairburn, (Eds.). *Eating disorders and obesity,* (pp. 289–293). New York: The Guilford Press.

Fairburn, C. G. (1995). Short-term psychological treatments for bulimia nervosa. In K. D. Brownell, & C. G. Fairburn, (Eds.). *Eating disorders and obesity,* (pp. 344–348). New York: The Guilford Press.

Fairburn, C. G., & Cooper, Z. (1993). The Eating Disorders Examination. In C. G. Fairburn & G. T. Wilson, (Eds). *Binge eating: nature, assessment, and treatment,* (pp. 317–360). New York: The Guildord Press.

Fairburn, C. G., & Walsh, B. T. (1995). Atypical eating disorders. In K. D. Brownell, & C. G. Fairburn, (Eds.). *Eating disorders and obesity,* (pp. 135–140). New York: The Guilford Press.

Fichter, M. M. (1995). Inpatient treatment of anorexia nervosa. In K. D. Brownell, & C. G. Fairburn, (Eds.). *Eating disorders and obesity,* (pp. 336–343). New York: The Guilford Press.

Flatt, J. P. (1993). Dietary fat, carbohydrate balance and weight maintenance. *Annals of the New York Academy of Sciences.* 683:122–140.

Food and Nutrition Board of the National Academy of Sciences, National Research Council. (1989). *Recommended Dietary Allowances,* (10th ed.). Washington, D.C.: National Academy Press.

Food and Nutrition Board, Institute of Medicine. (1995). *Weighing the Options: Criteria for Evaluating Weight-Management Programs.* Washington, D.C.: National Academy Press.

Foss, M. L. (1984). Exercise concerns and precautions for the obese. In J. Storlie & H. A. Jordan, (Eds.), *Nutrition and exercise in obesity management* (pp. 123–148). New York: Spectrum Books.

Fox, K. P. (1992). A clinical approach to exercise in the markedly obese. In T. A. Wadden T. B. Van Itallie, (Eds.). *Treatment of the Seriously Obese Patient,* (pp. 354–82). New York: The Guildford Press.

Garfinkel, P. E. (1995). Classification and diagnosis of eating disorders. In K. D. Brownell, & C. G. Fairburn, (Eds.). *Eating disorders and obesity,* (pp. 125–134). New York: The Guilford Press.

Garfinkel, L. (1985). Overweight and cancer. *Annals of Internal Medicine* 103, 1034.

Garner, D. M. (1995). Measurement of eating disorder psychopathology. In K. D. Brownell, & C. G. Fairburn, (Eds.). *Eating disorders and obesity,* (pp. 117–124). New York: The Guilford Press.

Giannini, A. J. (1993). A history of bulimia. in A. J. *Giannini & A. E. Slaby, (Eds.), The Eating Disorders* (pp. 18–21). New York: Springer-Verlag.

Goldbloom, D. S., & Kennedy, S. H. (1995). Medical complications of anorexia nervosa. In K. D. Brownell, & C. G. Fairburn, (Eds.). *Eating disorders and obesity,* (pp. 266–270). New York: The Guilford Press.

Goldstein, D. J. (1992). Beneficial health effects of modest weight loss. *International Journal of Obesity* 16, 397–415.

Gortmaker, S. L., Must, A., Perrin, J. M., & Dietz, W. H. (1993). Social and economic consequences of overweight in adolescence and young adulthood. *New England Journal of Medicine.* 329:1008–1012.

Graham, D.J., & Green L. (1997). Further cases of valvular heart disease associated with fenfluramine-phentermine [Letter to the editor]. *New England Journal of Medicine, 337,* 635.

Grilo, C. M., & Brownell, K. D. (1993). "Relapse: Why, How and What to Do About It." *Weight Control Digest* vol. 1, No. 3, 217–232.

Grundy, S. M. & Barneltt, J. P. (1990). Metabolic and health complications of obesity. In R. C. Bone, (Ed.). *Disease-a-month,* (vol. 36 pg. 643–731) St. Louis: C. V. Mosby Year Book.

Guy-Grand, B. (1992). Long-term pharmacological treatment of obesity.In Wadden, T. A. and Van Itallie, T. B. (Eds.). *Treatment of the Seriously Obese Patient,* (pp. 478–95). New York: The Guildford Press.

Gwinup, G. (1970). *Energetics: Your key to weight control.* Los Angeles: Sherbourne Press.

Heshka, S., & Heymsfield, S. B. (1995). Pharmacological treatment of obesity. In K. D. Brownell, & C. G. Fairburn, (Eds.). *Eating disorders and obesity,* (pp. 504–509). New York: The Guilford Press.

Hoek, H. W. (1995). The distribution of eating disorders. In K. D. Brownell, & C.G. Fairburn, (Eds.). *Eating disorders and obesity,* (pp. 207–211). New York: The Guilford Press.

Hubert, H. B., Feinlieb, M., McNamara, I. I., et. al. (1983). Obesity as an independent risk factor for heart disease: A 26-year follow-up of participants in the Framingham heart study. *Circulation,* 67, 968–977.

Irwin, E. G. (1993). A focused overview of anorexia nervosa and bulimia: part II—challenges of the practice of psychiatric nursing. *Archives of Psychiatric Nursing.* 7, 347–352.

Jeffrey, R., Wing, R., & French, S. (1992). Weight cycling and cardiovascular disease risk factors in obese men and women. *American Journal of Clinical Nutrition* 55, 641–644.

Jequier, E., & Felber, J. P. (1987). Indirect calorimetry. *Baillieres Cliniques Endocrinologie et Metabolism* 1(4), 911–935.

Jequier, E. (1990). Energy metabolism in obese patients before and after weight loss, and in patients who have relapsed. *International Journal of Obesity* 14 (suppl 1), 59–67.

Johnston, F. E. (1985). Health implications of childhood obesity. *Annals of Internal Medicine* 103, 1068.

Jordan, H. A., Levitz, L. S., & Kimbrell, G. M. (1976). *Eating is okay.* New York: Rawson Associates.

Kahn, H. S., Williamson, D. F. & Stevens, J. A. (1991). Race and weight change in US women: The roles of socioeconomic marital status. *American Journal of Public Health* 81, 319–323.

Kanders, B. S., & Blackburn, G. L. (1993). Very-low-calorie diets for the treatment of obesity. In G. L. Blackburn & B. S. Kanders (eds). *Obesity, pathophysiology, psychology, and treatment.* (pp. 197–216). New York: Chapman and Hall.

Kannel, W. B., Brand N., Skinner Jr., J. J., Dawber, R. F., & McNamara, P. M. (1967). The relationship of adiposity to blood pressure and development of hypertension: The Framingham Study. *Annals of Internal Medicine* 67, 48–59.

Kaplan. A. S., & Garfinkel, P. E. (1993). *Medical issues and the eating disorders: the interface.* New York: Brunner/Mazel Publishers.

Kato, I., Nomura, A., & Stemmetmann, G. N. (1992). Prospective study of clinical gallbladder disease and its association with obesity, physical activity, and other factors. *Digestive Diseases and Sciences* 37, 784–90.

Keys, A., Brozek, J. Henschel, A., Mickelsen, O., & Taylor, H. L. (1950). *The biology of human starvation.* Vol 1. Minneapolis: University of Minnesota Press.

Kocjan. D. K., & Giannini, A. J. (1993). The history of obesity. in A. J. Giannini & A. E. Slaby, (Eds.), *The Eating Disorders* (pp. 22–28). New York: Springer-Verlag.

Kral, J. G. (1995). Surgical interventions for obesity. In K. D. Brownell, & C. G. Fairburn, (Eds.). *Eating disorders and obesity,* (pp. 510–515). New York: The Guilford Press.

Kuczmarski, R. S., Flegal, K. M., Campbell, S. M., & Johnson, C. L. (1994). Increasing prevalence of overweight among U.S. adults: The National Health and Nutrition Examination Surveys, 1960 to 1991. *Journal of the American Medical Association.* 272, 205–211.

Lantingua, R. A., Amatruda, J. A., & Biddle, T. L. (1980). Cardiac arrhythmias associated with a liquid protein diet for the treatment of obesity. *New England Journal of Medicine* 303, 735–38.

Lanzola, A., Tagliabue, G., & Bozzi, G. (1991). Obesity, diet, and body temperature. *Annals of Nutrition and Metabolism* 35, 274–283.

Lakka, T. A., Venalainen, J. M., Rauramaa, R., Salonen, R., Tuomilehto, J., & Salonen J. T. Relation of leisure-time physical activity and cardiorespiratory fitness to the risk of acute myocardial infarction in men. (1994). *New England Journal of Medicine.* 330, 1549–54.

Lapidus, L., Bentgsson, C., Larsson, B., et. al. (1984). Distribution of adipose tissue and risk of cardiovascular disease and death: 12-year follow-up of participants in the population study of Gothenborg, Sweden. *British Medical Journal,* 289, 1257–1261.

Lee, I. M., Hsieh, C. C., & Parrenbarger, R. S. Jr. (1995). Exercise intensity and longevity in men. *Journal of the American Medical Association.* 273, 1179–1184.

Lee, I. M., & Paffenbarger, R. S. Jr. (1992). Quetelet's index and risk of colon cancer in college alumni. *Journal of the National Cancer Institute* 84, 1326–31.

Leibowitz, S. F. (1995). Central physiological determinants of eating behavior and weight. In K. D. Brownell, & C. G. Fairburn, (Eds.). *Eating disorders and obesity,* (pp. 3–7). New York: The Guilford Press.

Lew, E. A., & Garfinkel, L. (1979). Variations in mortality by weight among 750,000 men and women. *Journal of Chronic Diseases* 32, 563–576.

Lichtman, S. W., Pisarska, K., & Berman, E. R. (1992). Discrepancy between self-reported and actual calorie intake and exercise in obese subjects. *New England Journal of Medicine* 327, 1893–8.

Lissner, L., Odell, P. & D'Agostino, R. (1991). Variability of body weight and health outcomes in the Framingham population. *New England Journal of Medicine* 324, 1839–1844.

Manson, J. E., Colditz, G. A., Stampfer, M. J., et. al. (1990). A prospective study of obesity and risk of coronary heart disease in women. *New England Journal of Medicine* 322, 882–889.

Mark, E.J., Patalas, E.D., Chang, H.T., Evans, R.J., & Kessler, S.C. (1997). Fatal pulmonary hypertension associated with short-term use of fenfluramine and phentermine. *New England Journal of Medicine, 337,* 602–606.

Mattila, K., Haavisto, M. & Rajala, R. (1986). Body mass index and mortality in the elderly. *British Medical Journal* 292, 867–868.

McMahon, S. W., Macdonald, G. J., Bernstein, L., Andrews, G., & Blacket, R. B. (1985). A randomized controlled trial of weight reduction and metoprolol in the treatment of hypertension in young overweight patients. *Clinical Experimental Pharmacology and Physiology.* 12, 267–271.

Mickley, D. W. (1994) Medical aspects of anorexia and bulimia. In Kinoy, B. P. (Ed.) Eating disorders: new directions in treatment and recovery. New York: Columbian University Press.

Mitchell, J. E. (1995). Medical complications of bulimia nervosa. In K. D. Brownell, & C. G. Fairburn, (Eds.). *Eating disorders and obesity,* (pp. 271–277). New York: The Guilford Press.

Must, A., Jacques, P. F., Dallal, G. E., Bajema, C. J., & Dietz, W. H. (1992). Long-term morbidity and mortality of overweight adolescents: a follow-up of the Harvard Growth Study of 1922–1935. *New England Journal of Medicine.* 327:1350–1355.

National Heart, Lung, and Blood Institute, National Institutes of Health. (1993). *Second report of the expert panel on detection, evaluation, and treatment of high blood cholesterol in adults, (Adult Treatment Panel II).* NIH Publication No. 93–3095. Washington, D.C.: U.S. Government Printing Office.

National Heart, Lung and Blood Institute, National Institutes of Health. (1991). *Infomemo* Spring.

National Institute of Diabetes and Digestive and Kidney Diseases. (1993). *Understanding adult obesity.* Rockville, MD: National Institutes of Health NIH Publication No. 94–3680.

National Institutes of Health (1985). "National Institutes of Health Consensus Development Panel on the Health Implications of Obesity: National Institutes of Health Consensus Development Conference Statement" *Annals of Internal Medicine* 103, 1073–1077.

National Institutes of Health (1987). *Gallbladder Disease,* Bethesda, MD.

National Institutes of Health. (1993). *The fifth report of the Joint National Committee on Detection, Evaluation, and Treatment of High Blood Pressure.* Washington, D.C.: U.S. Government Printing Office. NIH Publication No. 93–1088.

National Institutes of Health Technology Assessment Conference. (1992). Methods for voluntary weight loss and control. *Annals of Internal Medicine* 116, 942–949.

National Research Council. (1989). *Diet and health: Implications for reducing chronic disease risk.* Washington, D.C.: National Academy Press.

National Institutes of Health Technology Assessment Conference Panel. (1992). Methods for voluntary weight loss and control. *Annals of Internal Medicine* 116, 942–9.

Obesity Update Newsletter (1993). Winter. Thorofare, New Jersey.

Osterman, J., Lin, T., Nankin, H. R., Brown, K. A., & Hornung, C. A. (1992). Serum cholesterol profiles during treatment of obese outpatients with a very low calorie diet: effects of initial cholesterol levels. *International Journal of Obesity* 16, 49–58.

Paffenbarger, R. S., Hyde, R. T., & Wing, A. L. (1993). The association of changes in physical-activity level and other lifestyle characteristics with mortality among men. *New England Journal of Medicine* 328, 358–45.

Palmer, R. L. (1995). Sexual abuse and eating disorders. In K. D. Brownell, & C. G. Fairburn, (Eds.). *Eating disorders and obesity,* (pp. 230–233). New York: The Guilford Press.

Pate, R. R., Pratt, M., & Blair, S. N. (1995). Physical activity and public health: a recommendation from the Centers for Disease Control and Prevention and the American College of Sports Medicine. *Journal of the American Medical Association.* 273, 402–407.

Perkins, K. A., Epstein, L. H., & Stiller, R. L. (1989). Acute effects of nicotine on resting metabolic rate in cigarette smokers. *American Journal of Clinical Nutrition* 50, 545–550.

Perri, M. G. Improving maintenance of weight loss following treatment by diet and lifestyle modification. In Wadden, T. A. and Van Itallie, T. B. (Eds.). *Treatment of the seriously obese patient.* (pp. 456–77). New York: The Guildford Press.

Perri, M. G., Nezv, A. M. & Viegener, B. J. (1992). *Improving the long-term management of obesity.* New York: John Wiley and Sons.

Perri, M. G., Sears, S. F. Jr & Clark, J. E. (1993). Strategies for improving maintenance of weight loss: Toward a continuing care model of obesity management. *Diabetes Care* 16, 200–9.

Peternelj-Taylor, C. A. (1989). The effects of patient weight and sex on nurses' perceptions: a proposed model of nurse withdrawal. *Journal of Advances in Nursing* 14, 744–54.

Peveler, R. C. (1995). Eating disorders and diabetes. In K. D. Brownell, & C. G. Fairburn, (Eds.). *Eating disorders and obesity,* (pp. 278–280). New York: The Guilford Press.

Polivy, J. (1996). Psychological consequences of food restriction. *Journal of the American Dietetic Association.* 96, 589–593.

Price, R. A., Stunkard, A. J. (1989). Commingling analysis of obesity in twins. *Human Heredity* 39, 121–35.

Ravussin, E. (1995). Energy expenditure and body weight. In K. D. Brownell, & C. G. Fairburn, (Eds.). *Eating disorders and obesity,* (pp. 32–37). New York: The Guilford Press.

Ravussin, E. (1993). Energy metabolism in obesity: Studies in the Pima Indians. *Diabetes Care* 16, 232–238.

Ravussin, E., Lillioja, S., & Knowler, W. C. (1988). Reduced rate of energy expenditure as a risk factor for body-weight gain. *New England Journal of Medicine* 318, 467–72.

Reichert, K. (1993) *Nutrition for recovery: eating disorders.* Boca Raton, FL: CRC Press, Inc.

Roberts, S. B., Savage, J., & Coward, W. A. (1988). Energy expenditure and intake in infants born to lean and overweight mothers. *New England Journal of Medicine* 318, 461–466.

Robison, J., Hoerr, S. L., & Strandmark, J. (1993). Obesity, weight loss, and health. *Journal of the American Dietetic Association* 93, 445–449.

Rosen, J. C. (1995). Assessment and treatment of body image disturbance. In K. D. Brownell, & C. G. Fairburn, (Eds.). *Eating disorders and obesity,* (pp.207–211). New York: The Guilford Press.

Rossouw, J. E., Lewis, B. & Rifkind, B. M. (1990). The value of lowering cholesterol after myocardial infarction. *New England Journal of Medicine* Oct 18, 1112–13.

Roubenoff, R., Klag, M. J. & Mead, L. A., et. al. (1991). Incidence and risk factors for gout in white men. *Journal of the American Medical Association* 266, 3004-7.

Sandvik, L., Erikssen, J., & Thaulow, E. (1993). Physical Fitness as a Predictor of Mortality Among Healthy, Middle-Aged Norwegian Men. *New England Journal of Medicine* 328, 533–7.

Schachter, S. (1971). Some extraordinary facts about obese humans and rats. *American Journal of Psychology,* 26, 129–144.

Schapiru, D. V., Kimar, N. B., & Lyman, G. H. (1990). Abdominal obesity and breast cancer risks. *Annals of Internal Medicine* 112, 182–186.

Schauer, P. R., Ramos, R. & Ghiatas, A. A., et. al. (1992). Virulent diverticular disease in young obese men. *American Journal of Surgery* 164, 443–46.

Schotte, D. E., & Stunkard, A. J. (1990). The effects of weight reduction on blood pressure in 301 obese patients. *Archives Internal Medicine.* 150:1701–1704.

Seim, H. C., & Holtmeier, K. B. (1992). Effects of a six-week, low-fat diet on serum cholesterol, body weight, and body measurements. *Family Practice Research Journal* 12, 411–419.

Sherry, B., Springer, D. A. & Connell, F. A. (1992). Short, thin, or obese?: Comparing growth indexes of children from high- and low-poverty areas. *Journal of the American Dietetic Association* 92, 1092–5.

Simonson, M., and Heilman, J. R. (1983). *The Complete University Medical Diet.* New York: Rawson Associates.

Sjostrom, L., Lissner, L., Larsson, B., et. al. (1994). SOS-Swedish obese subjects: an intervention study of obesity [abstract]. *International Journal of Obesity* 18 (suppl. 2):14.

Slaby, A. E., & Dwenger, R. (1993). History of anorexia nervosa. in A. J. Giannini & A. E. Slaby, (Eds.), *The Eating Disorders* (pp. 18–21). New York: Springer-Verlag.

Smith G. P., & Gibbs, J. (1995). Peripheral physiological determinants of eating and body weight. In K. D. Brownell, & C. G. Fairburn, (Eds.). *Eating disorders and obesity,* (pp. 8–12). New York: The Guilford Press.

Society of Actuaries and Association of Life Insurance Medical Directors of America. (1960). *1959 Build and Blood Pressure Study.* Chicago, IL: Society of Actuaries.

Society of Actuaries and Association of Life Insurance Medical Directors of America. (1980). *Build Study of 1979.* Chicago, IL: Society of Actuaries.

Stein, R. F. (1987). Comparison of self-concept of non-obese and obese university junior female nursing students. *Adolescence* 22, 77–90.

Stein, J. S., and Lowney, T. (1986). Obesity: The role of physical activity. In K. D. Brownell & J. T. Foreyt (Eds.), *Handbook of eating disorders* (pp. 145–158). New York: Basic Books.

Stephenson, J. N., Ohlrich, E. S., McClintock, J. H., Foster, S. W., Reinke, J. A., Allen, M. E., & Giles, G. M. (1988). The multidisciplinary team approach to the treatment of eating disorders in youth. In K. L. Clark, R. B. Parr, & W. P. Castelli, (Eds), *Evaluation and management of eating disorders: anorexia, bulimia, and obesity,* (pp. 261–278). Champaign, Illinois: Life Enhancement Publications.

Stuart, R. B., and Davis B. (1972). *Slim chance in a fat world: Behavioral control of obesity.* Champaign, IL: Research Press.

Stunkard, A.J. (1980). *Obesity.* Philadelphia: W. B. Saunders Company.

Stunkard, A. J. (1992). An overview of current treatment for obesity. In T. A. Wadden & T. B. Van Itallie, (Eds.). *Treatment of the Seriously Obese Patient.* New York: The Guildford Press.

Stunkard, A. J. (1995). Prevention of obesity. In K. D. Brownell, & C. G. Fairburn, (Eds.). *Eating disorders and obesity,* (pp. 572–576). New York: The Guilford Press.

The Surgeon General's report on nutrition and health (1988). U.S. Department of Health and Human Services. DHHS (PHS) Publication No. 88-50210. Washington, D.C.: U.S. Government Printing Office.

Task Force to Establish Weight Loss Guidelines. (1990). *Toward safe weight loss: recommendations for adult weight loss programs in Michigan.* East Lansing, MI: Michigan Health Council.

Tremblay, A., Despres, J. P., Maheux, J., et al. (1991). *Medical Science Sports and Exercise* 23, 1326–1331.

Tuschen, B. & Bents, H. (1995). Intensive brief inpatient treatment of bulimia nervosa. In K. D. Brownell, & C. G. Fairburn, (Eds.). *Eating disorders and obesity,* (pp. 354–360). New York: The Guilford Press.

U.S. Congress, House. (1990). *Deception and fraud in the diet industry, part I.* Hearing before the subcommittee on Regulation, Business Opportunities and Energy. Committee on Small Business. 101st Congress, 2nd Session. Washington, D.C.: Government Printing Office.

U.S. Department of Agriculture and Health and *Human Services. (1990). Nutrition and your health: Dietary guidelines for Americans,* (3rd ed.). Washington, D.C.: U.S. Government Printing Office.

U.S. Department of Agriculture and Health and Human Services. (1995). *Nutrition and your health: Dietary guidelines for Americans,* (4th ed.). Washington, D.C.: U.S. Government Printing Office.

U.S. Department of Agriculture, Human Nutrition Information Service. (1992). *Food guide pyramid: A guide to daily food choices,* Leaflet No. 572. Washington, D.C.: U.S. Government Printing Office.

U.S. Department of Health and Human Services. (1991). *Healthy people 2,000: National health promotion and disease prevention objectives.* DHHS (PHS) Publ. No. 91-50212. Public Health Service. Washington, D.C.: U.S. Government Printing Office.

Van Dale, D., Saris, W. H. M. & ten Hoor, F. (1990). Weight maintenance and resting metabolic rate 18-40 months after a diet/exercise treatment. *International Journal of Obesity* 14, 347–60.

Vandereycken, W. (1995). The families of patients with an eating disorder. In K. D. Brownell, & C. G. Fairburn, (Eds.). *Eating disorders and obesity,* (pp. 219–223). New York: The Guilford Press.

VanItallie, T. B., & Simopoulos, A. P. (1995) *Obesity: New directions in assessment and management.* Philadelphia: The Charles Press, Publishers.

Waaler, H. T. (1983). Weight and mortality: The Norwegian experience. *Acta Medica Scandinavica* 649, 1–55.

Wadden, T. A. (1995). Very-low-calorie diets: appraisal and recommendations. In K. D. Brownell, & C. G. Fairburn, (Eds.). *Eating disorders and obesity,* (pp. 484–490). New York: The Guilford Press.

Wadden, T. A., Sternberg, A. J., & Letizia K. A. (1989). Treatment of obesity by very low calorie diet, behavior therapy, and their combination: A five-year perspective. *International Journal of Obesity* 13, 39–46.

Wadden, T. A., & Stunkard, A. J. (1986). A controlled trial of very-low-calorie diet, behavior therapy, and their combination in the treatment of obesity. *Journal of Consultations in Clinical Psychology* 54, 482–488.

Walberg-Rankin, J. (1992). Utilizing exercise in the treatment of obesity. *Comprehensive Therapy* 18, 31–4.

Walsh, T. B. (1995). Pharmacotherapy of eating disorders. In K. D. Brownell, & C. G. Fairburn, (Eds.). *Eating disorders and obesity,* (pp. 207-211). New York: The Guilford Press.

Ward, E. M. (1994). Winners or losers? EN reviews the top weight-loss programs. *Environmental Nutrition.* 17:1, 3–5.

Weinsier, R. L. (1995). Clinical assessment of obese patients. In K. D. Brownell, & C. G. Fairburn, (Eds.). *Eating disorders and obesity,* (pp. 463–468). New York: The Guilford Press.

Wilfley, D. E., & Rodin, J. (1995). Cultural influences on eating disorders. In K. D. Brownell, & C. G. Fairburn, (Eds.). *Eating disorders and obesity,* (pp. 78–82). New York: The Guilford Press.

Willard, M. D. (1991). Obesity: types and treatments. *American Family Physician* 43, 2099–108.

Williamson, D. A. (1990). *Assessment of eating disorders.* New York: Pergamon Press.

Williamson, D. F. (1995). Prevalence and demographics of obesity. In K. D. Brownell, & C. G. Fairburn, (Eds.). *Eating disorders and obesity,* (pp. 391–395). New York: The Guilford Press.

Wilson, G. T. (1995). Behavioral approaches to the treatment of obesity. In K. D. Brownell, & C. G. Fairburn, (Eds.). *Eating disorders and obesity,* (pp. 479–483). New York: The Guilford Press.

Winick, M. (1985). *Your personalized health profile: Choosing the diet that's right for you.* New York: William Morrow and Company.

Wolf, A. M., & Colditz, G. A. (1994). The cost of obesity: The US perspective. *Pharmaco Economics* 5 (Suppl 1), 34–37.

Wood, P. D., Stefanick, M. L., Dreon, D. M., Frey-Hewitt, D. B., Garay, S. C., Williams, P. T., Superko, H. R., Fortmann, S. P., Albers, J. J., & Vranizan, K. M. (1988). Changes in plasma lipids and lipoproteins in overweight men during weight loss through dieting as compared with exercise. *New England Journal of Medicine* 319, 1173–1179.

World Health Organization. (1992). *IDC-10 classification of mental and behavioral disorders: clinical descriptions and diagnostic guidelines.* Geneva: World Health Organization.

Young, T., Palta, M., Dempsey, J., Skatrud, J., Weber, S., & Dabr, S. (1993). The occurrence of sleep-disordered breathing among middle-aged adults. *New England Journal of Medicine* 328, 1230–1235.

Zelasko, C. J. (1995). Exercise for weight loss: what are the facts? *Journal of the American Dietetic Association.* 95, 1414–1417.

INDEX

PRETEST KEY

1.   c   Chapter 1
2.   a   Chapter 1
3.   c   Chapter 2
4.   b   Chapter 2
5.   a   Chapter 3
6.   d   Chapter 3
7.   c   Chapter 4
8.   b   Chapter 4
9.   d   Chapter 5
10. d   Chapter 5
11. a   Chapter 6
12. b   Chapter 6
13. d   Chapter 7
14. c   Chapter 7
15. b   Chapter 8
16. c   Chapter 8
17. c   Chapter 9
18. c   Chapter 9
19. c   Chapter 9
20. d   Chapter 10
21. a   Chapter 10
22. c   Chapter 11
23. b   Chapter 11
24. d   Chapter 12
25. d   Chapter 13

Notes